# Healthcare Performance Measurement

## Systems Design and Evaluation

**Also available from ASQ Quality Press**

*The Effectiveness of CQI in Health Care:*
*Stories from a Global Perspective*
Vahé Kazandjian, editor

*The Handbook for Managing Change*
*in Health Care*
*ASQ Health Care Series*
Chip Caldwell, editor

*CQI and the Renovation of an American Health*
*Care System: A Culture Under Construction*
Sister Mary Jean Ryan, FSM, and William P. Thompson

*Stop Managing Costs: Designing Health Care*
*Organizations Around Core Business Systems*
James P. Mozena, Charles E. Emerick, and Steven C. Black

*How to Lower Health Care Costs by Improving Health Care*
*Quality: Results-Based Continuous Quality Improvement*
M. Daniel Sloan

*Statistical Quality Control Using Excel*
Steven M. Zimmerman and Marjorie L. Icenogle

*Mapping Work Processes*
Dianne Galloway

*Creativity, Innovation, and Quality*
Paul E. Plsek

*101 Good Ideas: How to Improve Just About Any Process*
Karen Bemowski and Brad Stratton, editors

To request a complimentary catalog of ASQ Quality Press
publications, call 800-248-1946.

# Healthcare Performance Measurement

## Systems Design and Evaluation

**Vahé A. Kazandjian, Ph.D., MPH**
*President*
Center for Performance Sciences, Inc.
Lutherville, Maryland USA
and
Adjunct Associate Professor
The Johns Hopkins University
School of Hygiene and Public Health
Baltimore, Maryland USA

Gallup Senior Scientist
The Gallup Organization
Princeton, New Jersey USA

**Terry R. Lied, Ph.D.**
Director, Indicator Development
MHA—The Association of Maryland Hospitals
and Health Systems
Quality Indicator Project®
Lutherville, Maryland USA

ASQ Quality Press
Milwaukee, Wisconsin

*Healthcare Performance Measurement: Systems Design and Evaluation*
Vahé A. Kazandjian and Terry R. Lied

**Library of Congress Cataloging-in-Publication Data**

Kazandjian, Vahe A.
  Healthcare performance measurement : systems design and evaluation
  / authors, Vahe A. Kazandjian, Terry Lied.
      p.    cm.
  ISBN 0-87389-436-7 (hardcover : alk. paper)
  1. Medical care—United States—Evaluation.    2. Medical care—
United States—Quality control.    3. Outcome assessment (Medical
care)    I. Lied, Terry, 1947–    .  II. Title.
  [DNLM:    1. Quality Indicators, Health Care.    2. Outcome Assessment
(Health Care)—methods.    W 84.1 K23h 1999]
  RA399.A3K36    1999
  362.1'068'5—dc21
  DNLM/DLC
  for Library of Congress                                                99–10898
                                                                                            CIP

© 1999 by ASQ

10 9 8 7 6 5 4 3 2

ISBN 0-87389-436-7

Acquisitions Editor:  Ken Zielske

Project Editor:  Annemieke Koudstaal

Production Coordinator:  Shawn Dohogne

ASQ Mission: The American Society for Quality advances individual and organizational performance excellence worldwide by providing opportunities for learning, quality improvement, and knowledge exchange.

*Attention: Bookstores, Wholesalers, Schools and Corporations:*
ASQ Quality Press books, videotapes, audiotapes, and software are available at quantity discounts with bulk purchases for business, educational, or instructional use. For information, please contact ASQ Quality Press at 800-248-1946, or write to ASQ Quality Press, P.O. Box 3005, Milwaukee, WI 53201-3005.

To place orders or to request a free copy of the ASQ Quality Press Publications Catalog, including ASQ membership information, call 800-248-1946. Visit our web site at http://www.asq.org.

Printed in the United States of America

♾ Printed on acid-free paper

**American Society for Quality**

# ⊞ASQ™

Quality Press
611 East Wisconsin Avenue
Milwaukee, Wisconsin 53202
Call toll free 800-248-1946
http://www.asq.org
http://standardsgroup.asq.org

To our wives, Janet and Deborah, and our children
Ani, Gregory, and Christopher

# Contents

**Chapter 4**
**Evaluating the Construct of a Performance**

# Contributors to Field Stories

**Regina Coady**
*Director of Qualitive Initiatives*
Health Care Corporation of St. John's
Newfoundland, Canada

**Brian T. Collopy, M.B.B.S.**
*Director, Department of Colon and Rectal Surgery*
St. Vincent's Hospital
Melbourne, Australia

**Cathy Davis**
*Director of Health Record Services*
Mount Sinai Hospital
Toronto, Ontario, Canada

**Nancy C. Gault, BScN, MHSA**
*Research and Development*
Canadian Council on Health Services Accreditation
Ottawa, Canada

**Arlene N. Hayne, R.N., D.S.N., B.S.N.**
*Corporate Director, Quality Management*
Baptist Health System, Inc.
Birmingham, Alabama

**Michael J. Hill, M.Ed.**
*President*
Foundation for Healthy Communities
New Hampshire Hospital Association
Concord, New Hampshire

**Nancy Kelly**
*Assistant Executive Director, Patient Services*
Renfrew Victoria Hospital
Renfrew, Ottawa, Canada

**Mark Mycyk**
*Quality Associate*
St. Michael's Hospital
Toronto, Ontario, Canada

**Rachel M. Rowe, R.N., M.S.**
*Executive Vice President*
Foundation for Healthy Communities
New Hampshire Hospital Association
Concord, New Hampshire

**Joanne W. Williams, Ph.D.**
*Epidemiologist*
The Australian Council on Healthcare Standards
Victoria, Australia

# Foreword

"And stand together: yet not too near together
For the pillars of the temple stand apart
And the oak tree and the cypress
grow not in each other's shadow."
*Gibran, The Prophet*

We wrote this book after 12 years of experience in the design of performance profiling strategies (PPS). The Maryland Hospital Association's Quality Indicator Project (QI Project ®) is our model. It is the single most widely used performance measurement project in healthcare in the United States and is also used in 10 other countries. We wanted to share with those aiming to build an indicator-focused profiling strategy the issues we faced and how we addressed those issues. In our minds that has been the *oak tree* Gibran talked about. We wanted to find the *cypress*.

The cypress, in our minds, is the psychometric discipline. This discipline is not only a systematic science of inquiry and evaluation; it is the discipline most suitable to addressing issues of social significance. Today, *accountability* is the main reason for the *report card mentality* in conveying to various audiences how well an institution is performing. When providing pattern and trend analysis to support statements about performance profiles, the report card is becoming a preoccupation of many healthcare organizations. It is, therefore, natural to think about a healthcare PPS as having a pronounced social obligation. This social obligation is, in fact, reinforced by formal requirements for demonstrating good performance by accrediting agencies, regulatory bodies, and employer groups. Institutions that delay in adopting measurement systems risk loss of credibility, market share, and possibly their accreditation status.

But we still wonder how close together the oak tree and cypress should grow. We wonder if the measurement systems, in order to thrive within a performance profile demonstration strategy, need fertile soil and open space to grow deep roots, to branch out, and to weather the winds of change facing our field. Or, we wonder if the cypress and the oak tree need to be close in order to create and sustain a harmonious twosome whereby each will grow, supporting each other when the terrain is dry, weathering the winds of change together, and, together, in their shadow, nurturing new trees.

This book is a unique attempt to address some of these questions. Do we have the answers? To provide further support to the targets of our inquiry, we asked colleagues from the United States, Australia, and Canada to share with us their local, regional, and national initiatives addressing these very questions. We present these national issues as stories from the field in a section by itself.

When we put down our pens and looked at the pages we filled with our wondrous looks, our concrete examples, our review of methods, our theories of groups and institutions, and our stories from the field, we realized that we ourselves were at a turning point. We knew that measuring performance and demonstrating the merits of a performance profile is not a research project anymore. Rather, based upon the past decade's accumulated experience, there was enough theory and practice to establish a discipline! And why not? If the work in the United States and abroad in the area of indicators, measurement systems, and evaluation of outcomes is to culminate in a comprehensive performance profiling strategy, then it needs to become a discipline.

We look forward to the day when indicators will have a common design; when a clinical rate will be evaluated within the context of cost, resource utilization, and satisfaction; and when a report card will tell its specific audiences if the provider was acceptably accountable to them. Until that day, we will wonder, as perhaps you will, if the oak tree and the cypress should grow in each other's shadow.

# Acknowledgments

The authors would like to express their appreciation to Laura Pimentel of the Maryland Hospital Association for organizing the preparation of the manuscript and for keeping us on track for promised deadlines for three books in a row. The authors would also like to express their appreciation to Dana Maher, graduate student in Epidemiology at Johns Hopkins University, Baltimore, Maryland for her comments on an earlier version of the manuscript. And, last, we thank Cal Pierson, President of MHA: The Association of Maryland Hospitals and Health Systems, for his continuing support of scholarly work.

# List of Figures

# 1

# Principles of the Genesis of the Design of a Performance Measurement System

## INTRODUCTION

We are all interested in performance. The performance that we associate with providers of social services is becoming increasingly noticeable in its immediacy and importance across cultures and geography. Healthcare, which encompasses medicine and public health, is now at the center of social attention. At the beginning of the millennium, all countries and health systems are faced with the same dilemma: How much *healthcare* should people receive, when should they receive it, and at what cost?

Much has been echoed in the literature about the importance of understanding performance. Borrowing from industrial models of production, where efficiency of production is paramount, many have proposed that healthcare be viewed under the same magnifying glass as the production of other social goods. In doing so, it is natural to suppose that performance measures are equally applicable in industry and medicine. A number of initiatives, both in the United States and abroad, have explored the feasibility of indicators and demonstrated that the magnitude of an event, the patterns of its happening, and its longitudinal profile affect institutions, providers, and recipients! We would like to explore the genesis of the design of a performance measurement system based on the following principles that we will follow throughout this book.

- Indicators have to indicate. We have found it difficult to find true indicators when it comes to healthcare performance measurement.

- Performance indicators do not measure performance, people do. This is a fundamental premise whereby we will explore the importance of training the user rather than landing the measures.

- While measurement can be global, evaluation is always local. Thus, the value one places upon the measured profile is expected to be affected by local philosophies and expectations.

- Performance can be described through a step-wise paradigm of measurement, evaluation, and monitoring. These premises underlie all performance measurement design. If a shift in mentality, a shift in performance level, a shift in expectations, and a shift in the application of social and medical sciences are not undertaken in earnest, then designing a performance measurement system remains an academic exercise, incapable of fulfilling the goal of accountability.

- Institutional performance should not only be measured at the level of the institution; it should extend and be reflected in the health status and functionality of patients subsequent to their hospitalization (or receipt of other services).

It seems that performance measurement systems are on the agenda of every regulatory group, every institution, and practically all government bodies involved in providing or regulating healthcare systems both in the United States and internationally. It is, perhaps, easier to understand who has the authority and capability to develop a performance measurement system at the international level than it is in the United States. In countries where the governmental system has a ministry of health, the activities related to developing, applying, and monitoring various aspects of the performance system fall under the aegis of the ministry of health. In the developing world, such ministries have the interest and sometimes the capability to bring in experts from the proven record *fields* of public health, medicine, and hospital administration to help in measuring and rewarding performance. Although traditional public health activities fall under the aegis of ministries of health, it is not clear if performance measurement that cuts across clinical and public health dimensions can be naturally hosted within the ministry of health. Such an observation is not unexpected. The literature, primarily from Western European countries and the United States, has debated the importance of measuring performance as a clinical paradigm.

The changing of mind-sets regarding the importance of bringing public health and medicine together is relatively new, as is thinking about the continuum of care rather than the hospitalization episode. Acceptance of the interaction of prevention and cure (as well as the interactions of social dimensions of medicine and public health applications) may be more commonplace in countries where ministries of health have significant power over providers of care. It is a challenging idea since in many countries the concept of performance measurement is just becoming accepted.

The usefulness of performance measurement, which entails financial accountability and responsiveness to the community, is slowly being acknowledged in many countries. Perhaps additional effort should be spent with countries that have the necessary infrastructure and the mind-set to view both public health and medicine as a seamless continuum aimed at providing a social service. When the system is similar to the U.S. or the British system, there can be numerous variations on the theme of who should develop or host the application of a performance measurement system. Academic institutions have shown some interest in the matter. However, given the nature of academia and the inherent time frame necessary to conduct research and publish findings, academic settings have not played a major role in the development or the application of performance measurement systems. Rather, the impetus for such systems has come from providers and payers of services in an attempt to determine how they are doing compared to their competitors. Academic expertise has been widely employed during the development of the evaluation of performance measurement systems. However, the questions addressing the need for such systems have been answered in a direction suggesting a commitment to immediate application. As a result, performance measurement systems have found a happy environment in a multitude of professional institutions and trade associations.

## THE PHILOSOPHICAL BASIS OF PERFORMANCE MEASUREMENT

Each of us tends to think we see things as they are, that we are objective. But this is not the case. We see the world, not as it is, but as we are—or, as we're conditioned to see it. When we open our mouths to describe what we see, we in effect describe ourselves, our perceptions, our paradigms. (Covey, 1989)

Performance measurement is based on assumptions rooted in science as well as philosophy. Some of these assumptions have been altered during the twentieth century, due to new approaches to understanding measurement phenomena such as Heisenberg's *Uncertainty Principle* (Brennan, 1997) and Einstein's *Special Theory of Relativity* (Davies, 1995). The Heisenberg Principle, in brief, states that the act of measurement, itself, alters the event being measured. Einstein's Theory of Relativity proposes that distance and time are not independent of the motion of the observer, and, hence, their measurement is *relative*.

### Assumptions of Performance Measurement

We propose five assumptions underlying performance measurement, which include both uncertainty and relativity (see Figure 1.1). Our five assumptions are based on a *worldview* that is not shared by all people, but this *worldview* is shared by virtually all of the twentieth century scientists. Our measurement assumptions are as follows:

- Measurement is relative in the sense that it is never independent of our perceptions, our instrumentation, and our position in time and space. This assumption implies that measurement in healthcare is never exact nor is it ever completely independent of the observer.

- There is a state of uncertainty in the measurement of any event. This uncertainty frequently reflects *randomness* which, while problematic to measurement, is not the predominant state of reality. This assumption implies that despite some inherent uncertainty, the measurement of performance in healthcare is often useful and scientifically valid.

- There is an objective reality independent of the human mind. This implies that performance is *real* and there are *real* differences in healthcare performers.

- The world has order and predictability. It follows that healthcare and its measurement obey the laws of nature—which are predictable.

- *Reality* is measurable; it can be quantified. We can validly assign numbers to events that reflect reality in healthcare.

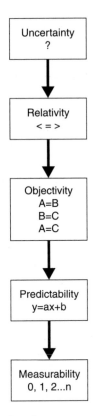

**Figure 1.1.** Five assumptions of performance measurement.

We begin our investigations of performance measurement by assuming an objective reality—a reality independent of the human mind. Beauty may be in the eye of the beholder, but there is still an objective reality—or, at least, we must assume there is if we are to discuss performance measurement in a scientific fashion. Just as important as the assumption of an objective reality, for our purposes, is the assumption that we can validly measure that objective reality.

### Accuracy and Validity

To a large extent, the accuracy and validity of measurement depends on the competence of the measure's filters—the measure's ability to eliminate the irrelevant—just as the mind depends on the competence of its filters for healthy functioning. When we measure, we restrict our senses, attention, and observations to a set of specific phenomena under special conditions; we filter *irrelevant* happenings, events, and phenomena. In healthcare, as in any discipline, we often suspend time when we measure events. Therefore, while the events are usually continuous, the measurements are usually discontinuous.

At best, we measure at intervals when we assess performance—*a type of sampling of reality.* While it is true that we may capture all of the cases of interest for a specific time period in our measurements, the measures do not provide real-time assessments of performance. Those assessments are periodic or sporadic; they can never be completely continuous.

## ANALYSIS AND INTERPRETATION

Performance measurement is of little consequence if interpretation and analysis of data do not accompany it. The analysis and interpretation of data can be made by the performance measurement system, itself, by the users, or by both users and the system. Performance measurement systems vary in the level of analysis and interpretation of data that they provide to their users. Some systems consider interpretation and analysis, forms of user-education, as integral to their *holistic* approach to performance measurement. Other systems concentrate on providing data at various levels of detail and sophistication and let interpretation primarily up to the user.

What is best: Present the data and let users make their own interpretation or offer analysis and interpretation as part of the performance measurement *package*? Audience sophistication is obviously a factor in this decision, but sometimes the audience varies greatly in terms of its background, knowledge, and experience in healthcare and measurement. A solid healthcare background does not guarantee an understanding of statistical concepts inherent in performance measurement and its interpretation. On the other hand, statistical knowledge does not equate with the ability to interpret the data of performance measurement if clinical knowledge is lacking.

To a large extent, the relative emphasis on analysis and interpretation depends on the objectives of the performance measurement system and its intended audience. An audience of physicians obviously has different data and analytic requirements than an audience of consumers. If any generality can be made here, it is that the design of a performance measurement system must be appropriate to the intended audience of that system, whether it is providers, consumers, payers, or regulators. One size may not fit all.

# WHAT IS MEASURABLE
## vs. WHAT IS IMPORTANT

A man saw Nasrudin searching for something on the ground. "What have you lost, Mulla?" He asked. "My key," said Nasrudin. So the man went down on his knees too, and they both looked for it. After a time, the other man asked: "Where exactly did you drop it?" "In my own house," said Nasrudin. "Then why are you looking here," said the other man. "There is more light here than inside my own house," said Nasrudin. (Shah, 1972)

As this Sufi story illustrates, it is human nature to conduct one's searches in an illuminated area, even if the object of one's search cannot be found there. Similarly, in performance measurement there appears to be a tendency to measure what is readily measurable, regardless of whether or not the thing measured is what is most important. What is most likely to be measured is usually what is most readily collected, quantified, and reported. The U.S. Health Care Financing Administration (HCFA) hospital mortality studies in the mid 1980s are a poignant reminder of how large-scale efforts to provide comparative outcomes data may find it difficult to avoid this pitfall (for example, Moskowitz, 1994). The HCFA studies used non-risk-adjusted mortality data as a proxy for performance in hospitals, making the data available to the public without appropriate caveats to accompany their release. The result was considerable public uproar based on flawed interpretations and comparisons. Unfortunately, such occurrences are common in most disciplines in which outcomes are measured.

There are a few disciplines or occupations, if you prefer, in which there is an inherently close association between what is measurable and what is important—what truly matters. A good illustration is in the arena of sports; both individual and team performance are quite measurable in sports vocations or avocations. In baseball, for example, individual performance (outcomes) can be readily assessed using batting averages, pitcher's earned run averages, fielding averages, and so on. In effect, these are all rates. Team performance is also measured by a rate: team *performance* = *total wins/total games*. Unlike baseball and many other sports, what is measurable in healthcare is often remote from what is most important; frequently, there are no direct measures of the most important outcomes such as there are in team performance. If it is the overall health status of the patient that matters—or, at least, what matters most—then the trick is to develop a valid measure of health status that is also conceptually and empirically tied to the healthcare that the patient receives.

In healthcare, outcomes are usually chosen that reflect a compromise between what can be measured and what is most important. For example, one common clinical outcomes measure is infection rates (nosocomial or surgical wound). When a patient undergoes surgery or hospitalization, is it the avoidance of these infections that is most important or the overall outcome of the surgery? We think that what matters most to patients is their improvement in health status or functioning as a result of the care they receive (the *ultimate outcome*), not their avoidance of infection when receiving care (the *immediate outcome*).

## IMMEDIATE, INTERMEDIATE, AND ULTIMATE OUTCOMES

We suggest that it is useful to view performance outcomes as immediate, intermediate, and ultimate (Donabedian, 1973). Immediate outcomes often concern adverse health—related events while ultimate outcomes involve potentialities for human health and functioning. Intermediate outcomes are somewhere between the two extremes: they do not reflect adverse events as an immediate consequence of the healthcare intervention nor do they reflect what matters most to the patient or the patient's guardian—why the intervention was sought in the first place. To avoid any misunderstanding, we are not saying that immediate and intermediate outcomes are not important to patients or their guardians; they are just not as important as ultimate outcomes. Patients are not always aware of the threats of poor immediate outcomes to their long-term health or well being. They or their guardians, however, are usually aware of why they are seeking medical care.

## PERFORMANCE MEASUREMENT SYSTEMS IN COMBINATION

Many times a single performance measurement system, while useful and cost-beneficial, will not meet all the needs of a healthcare facility. While a few performance measurement systems are relatively comprehensive or *integrated*—encompassing diverse aspects of performance such as financial, clinical, administrative, health status, and patient satisfaction data—

most concentrate on one area of measurement. Such *singular-focused* performance measurement systems may not serve all the measurement needs of a healthcare organization. The usual situation is that different departments of a healthcare facility have different concerns: clinical departments want clinical data, financial departments want financial data, and so on. Occasionally, and this seems to be an increasing phenomenon, a department or individuals are interested in an integrated approach to performance measurement—perhaps by combining the various components of cost, quality, and access into some global assessment of performance.

Whether healthcare facilities should attempt to recruit a performance measurement system that is all or nearly *all-inclusive* is a personal or organizational decision. If such a system is available and it satisfies the needs of the organization, then it may make good sense to consider such a system—given that it is affordable, will be around for a while, and so on. The disadvantage of such a strategy, however, is that if it backfires, there is no *bonafide* performance measurement until the system is replaced.

A more cautious approach to meeting the needs of comprehensive performance measurement, instead of choosing one all-encompassing system, is to select two or more performance measurement systems. One system can meet the need for clinical assessment, a second, for financial assessment, a third, for patient satisfaction. For example, given the state of the art, this is the usual situation faced by most healthcare organizations, whether they like it or not. The linkage and networking of disparate forms of healthcare data is still embryonic, even though many of the current computer software technologies can theoretically handle this challenge of integration. We are swiftly moving from a paper-based to an electronic, media-based world. The remnants of this paper-based world, one in which such linkages were impossible, are still preventing the complete emergence of this new informatics order. However, the trend is clear and the outcome seems inevitable due, at least in part, to the increased demand for the timely transport of vast amounts of data and information. The revolutionary nature of these requirements and their effects on the human psyche are eloquently expressed by Birkerts (1994). In a cogent collection of essays, he laments on the decline, if not demise, of the print medium, as we have come to know it, and its replacement by electronic media. For example, he states:

> We require swift and obedient tools with vast capacities for moving messages through networks. As the tools proliferate, however, more and

more of what we do involves network interaction. The processes that we created to serve our evolving needs have not only begun to redefine our experience, but they are fast becoming our new cognitive paradigm. It is ever more difficult for us to imagine how people ever got along before fax, e-mail, mobile phones, computer networks. (p. 153)

# PERFORMANCE MEASUREMENT AND THE GLOBAL HEALTHCARE ENVIRONMENT

Performance measurement in healthcare has gained momentum in the United States in recent years for several reasons. Perhaps the most important reason for this increased momentum is the emergence of *managed care* and its concomitant impact on cost controls and the quality of care. While the jury may still be out on whether or not *managed care* will increase or decrease overall quality of care, it is clear that its emergence has led to calls for new forms of accountability, spurring the development of performance measures and systems of measurement.

Outside the United States, performance measurement also appears to be getting more emphasis these days, although current measurement systems are generally more embryonic abroad than in the United States. Performance measurement systems that were developed in the United States and have a lengthy history are now being applied outside the United States, including Canada, Europe, and Asia[1]. The applicability and utility of these measures on a worldwide basis is still being tested. Until performance measurement reaches the *critical mass* in terms of participants in these counties, it will be difficult to compare performance among providers unless data from U.S. providers can be used to form a basis for the comparisons. The question is: Are healthcare delivery, documentation, and reporting methods sufficiently similar in these European and Asian countries to allow comparisons with U.S. aggregate data? The question is largely rhetorical since few if any research studies have addressed this issue, perhaps due as much to conceptual difficulties in dealing with problems of definition as the obvious difficulties in obtaining the comparative performance data.

---

[1]For example, performance indicators developed by Maryland's Quality Indicator Project® are now being used in Japan, Taiwan, Portugal, Russia, Flanders, Austria, the Netherlands, the United Kingdom, and Canada.

# THE TYPOLOGY OF PERFORMANCE MEASURES

There is an abundance of measures used to assess performance in healthcare, including measures of structures (financial, staffing ratios), processes (clinical pathways and clinical protocols), and outcomes (inpatient mortality, patient satisfaction, and health status). There are also disease-specific measures and measures designed to risk or severity-adjust other measures. Various typologies of performance measures exist to deal with the myriad of performance measures. A review of some of the most prominent typologies may be helpful in forming an in-depth understanding of the dimensions of performance measurement.

## *JCAHO Typology*

In the United States, one of the most recent typologies for performance indicators is listed in the 1997 *National Library of Health Care Indicators*™ published by the Joint Commission on Accreditation of Health Care Organizations (JCAHO). The four generic categories of performance indicators in the JCAHO framework are

- Clinical Performance

- Health Status

- Satisfaction

- Administrative/Financial

This framework was established and validated by the JCAHO under the guidance of an external advisory group comprised of "nationally recognized experts in network performance measurement, purchasers, payers, and practitioners."[2] The JCAHO delineates the four categories of performance indicators through a series of *matrices*. The *domains of clinical performance*, along with their definitions, are appropriateness, availability, continuity, effectiveness, efficacy, efficiency, prevention/early detection, respect and caring, safety, and timeliness. In addition, in the JCAHO rubric, health status measures are based on nine factors or *health concepts* developed by the Medical Outcomes Trust.[3] Administrative/financial performance involves three general aspects: provider and service delivery, administrative and financial, and overall satisfaction.

---

[2]National Library of Health Indicators™, Joint Commission on Accreditation of Healthcare Organizations. Oakbrook Terrace, IL: 1997, p. 3.

[3]Medical Outcomes Trust. *How to Score the SF-36 Health Survey,* Boston: 1994.

## Conquest

A very different typology of performance measures preceded the development of CONQUEST 1.0 and 1.1 (AHCPR, 1997). The acronym, CONQUEST, stands for the *Computerized Needs-Oriented Quality Measurement Evaluation System,* a prototype system for collecting and evaluating clinical performance measures (CONQUEST 1.0, 1996).[4] CONQUEST is a project funded by the U.S. Federal Government's Agency for Health Care Policy and Research (AHCPR) and developed by the Center for Quality of Care Research and Education under the leadership of Dr. R. Heather Palmer at the Harvard School of Public Health and Mikilax and Company. CONQUEST includes two interlocking databases—a measure and a condition database. These two databases have an interface, which allows users to obtain summary information on approximately 1200 extant clinical performance measures (developed by various public- and private-sector organizations in the United States).

The AHCPR typology is well-suited for those interested in designing and/or evaluating performance measures and performance measurement systems. It is relatively simple in structure and easy to understand, yet it contains all the main elements of performance measures.

## HEDIS

A third typology is the *Health Employer Data Information Set,* also known as HEDIS®. HEDIS was initially developed by a cooperative group of health plans, large employers, and the National Committee for Quality Assurance (NCQA) to help employers in the United States understand what they were getting for their healthcare dollars. HEDIS allows health plans to compare their performance with other health plans, to track their own performance over time, and to compare their progress in meeting external goals such as those promulgated by the U.S. Public Health Services' Healthy People 2000 initiative. HEDIS has been evolving since the late 1980s, a time when healthcare purchasers and plans first joined forces to discuss measures that would allow them to hold health plans accountable for their services. HEDIS performance measures involve many public health issues including heart disease, cancer, smoking, diabetes, and asthma.

---

[4]*CONQUEST 1.0, Overview: A Computerized Needs-oriented Quality Measurement Evaluation System.* President and Fellows of Harvard College, 1996. (http://www.ahcpr.gov/qual/conqovrl.htm).

The HEDIS *typology* consists of various dimensions.

- Quality
- Satisfaction
- Access to services
- Utilization
- General plan management
- Financial measures

# THE LIFE CYCLE OF PERFORMANCE MEASURES

The development of performance measures is a process that is cyclical in nature (see Figure 1.2). One or two measures, perhaps, even an entire set of performance measures, will be developed, tested, and implemented. After implementation, there is usually a period of suspended judgment, not infrequently followed by a period of modification or revision. There is also the eventual decline followed by *obsolescence*; our performance measure has a beginning and an ending—a *life cycle*. Its conception guarantees its eventual end. The generativity and fruitfulness of the period between its *birth* and *death* is a function of the quality of its conceptual genes, how well it is nurtured, its medico-political environment, and sheer happenstance. We will focus here on the management or nurturing, if you prefer, of a measure's life cycle.

**Planning.** The processes in planning a new measure are not unlike those involved in *family planning*. The timing of the event must be just right. The measure must be introduced in an appropriate milieu or it will not thrive. Resources have to be available to nurture the measure, to bring it along in its infancy. These resources literally include people who *care* about the measure—individuals who have a special interest in seeing it develop and reach its potential.[5]

Materialistic provisions for the new measure must also be planned. The measure must be properly packaged (clothed) to make it pleasing and to protect it from the elements during periods of vulnerability.[6] Its transport needs

---

[5]The authors are aware of instances when a new project or measure was said to be his or her *baby*. The readers may also have had such experiences.

[6]This reasoning is less farfetched than it may seem at first: measures must be clothed and housed. This clothing can include paper or electronic media materials—CDs diskettes, etc.

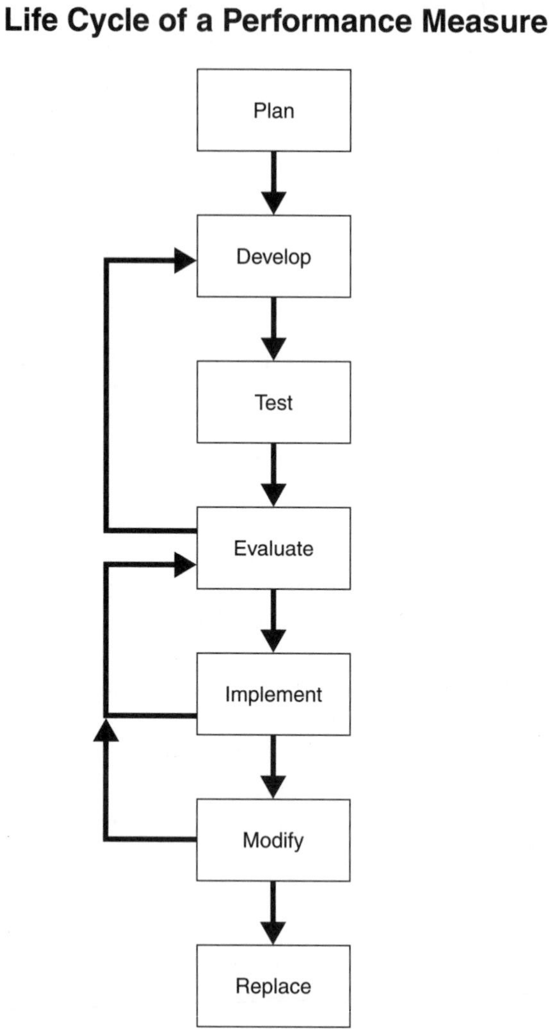

## Life Cycle of a Performance Measure

```
        ┌──────────┐
        │   Plan   │
        └────┬─────┘
             │
             ▼
   ┌───►┌──────────┐
   │    │ Develop  │
   │    └────┬─────┘
   │         │
   │         ▼
   │    ┌──────────┐
   │    │   Test   │
   │    └────┬─────┘
   │         │
   │         ▼
   └────┌──────────┐
        │ Evaluate │
   ┌───►└────┬─────┘
   │         │
   │         ▼
   │    ┌──────────┐
   │    │Implement │
   ▲    └────┬─────┘
   │         │
   │         ▼
   │    ┌──────────┐
   └────│  Modify  │
        └────┬─────┘
             │
             ▼
        ┌──────────┐
        │ Replace  │
        └──────────┘
```

**Figure 1.2.**   Steps in the management of the *Life Cycle* of a performance
measure.

must be planned (electronic media, internet, mail). Ultimately, in planning
the risks of survival during the measure's infancy must be evaluated.

**Developing.**   This is accomplished during the conceptual (or conception)
phase in the life cycle of a measure. The conceptual stage is important in
providing the right mix of genes for the measure; these genes are a kind of

blueprint, model, or, if you prefer, paradigm. The potential for the measure is set at this stage or, at least, its limitations are set here. Will it *measure up* to the demands placed upon it during its life span: will it be dependable (reliable), will it be useful (valid), will it handle adversity (risk-adjustment), will it be self-supporting, will it not demand too much attention, will it be fruitful (heuristic)? These traits are influenced by the measure's genetic underpinnings, the model or paradigm upon which it is based.

**Testing.** Testing occurs during the measure's formative stages— particularly prominent during its childhood, adolescence, and early adulthood. In fact, testing occurs throughout the measure's life span, but it has less ability to affect the development of the measure at later stages in its life. Testing can be done with the goal of improving the measure or to determine its potentialities and limitations. The results of the testing are used to evaluate the measure. That is, testing can be done for therapeutic and evaluative purposes.

**Evaluating.** Before the measure is ready to do what it was designed to do, there comes the inevitable assessment. The measure is well into its puberty now. Clearly, the concern is not only with its temporal blemishes but also with the likelihood of its ultimate worthiness. This is the most painful period for the measure's developers. It is a period that frequently involves soul-searching and second-guessing. Should more time have been spent in working with the measure during its formative stages? Perhaps there was some flaw in its genetic structure—a faulty paradigm or a mutated conceptualization. Perhaps it was exposed to toxic agents in its formative stages, arresting its development and posing serious limitations on its potentialities. Such second-guessing and soul-searching are unlikely to improve the measure; they are, however, likely to divert declining energies from the measure's rehabilitation, if that is an appropriate course of action.

Evaluating is deciding. At this point, there are at least four possibilities: implement, send the measure back for some readjustment or *rehab,* put the measure in layaway, a kind of limbo state, or scrap it. That is, one either sends the measure along to make its way, decides it needs more refinement, does nothing for the time being, or calls it a day. Layaway may be the least preferred course of action. The measure can still consume resources while it is in this state, even though it is generating no return or value. At least if it's scrapped, no more damage can be done—no more depletion of valuable resources; no more seemingly endless dialogue over the merits of the measure; no more rationalizations.

**Implementing.**   Implementation is, in effect, the real test of the measure. It is done during the *adult stage* of the measure. How will the measure fare under load conditions and real-life circumstances? Will it be useful, generative, cost-effective and have longevity? Will it be expensive to implement, short-lived, and yield little or no return? The measure may be implemented in spite of flaws, either known or unknown at the time of implementation. Known shortcomings are probably easier to handle than unanticipated ones, since the latter are less amenable to planning. Every measure has limitations and is flawed in the sense that it cannot meet all performance measurement needs of all users. These limitations have to be accepted if the measure is to be of any value to its users.

**Modifying.**   At least some modification (revision) is generally needed by the time the performance measure enters its midlife. The shiny new measure is beginning to lose its luster and it is facing its midlife crisis. The bloom has worn off, and adjustments must be made if the measure is to continue to be useful and generative. This stage is a test of the character and more enduring qualities of the measure. Does it have enough depth of character (reliability, validity) so that some adjustments involving an outlay of resources are warranted in preserving it or even enhancing its value? Most performance measures that have reached this stage have proved their dependability and usefulness and warrant some revision and repairs. Those showing just enough potential to justify implementation earlier are less likely to survive this *midlife* crisis. In actuality, more than one period of modification may be involved in salvaging a measure that is showing mid—life wear. Modification, then, becomes an iterative process with an eventual wind-down. This inevitable winding-down signals in the stage of obsolescence and the possible need for replacement.

**Replacing.**   Inexorably, a performance measure reaches a period of decline followed by its obsolescence. When mass supplants energy in a performance measure—when the measure begins to crumble under its own weight—it is time to be replaced. In fact, it is past time: the measure should have been forced into retirement before reaching this stage. Unfortunately, retirement like death comes too early or too late, and, we suspect, with performance measures, the latter is more customary than the former.

Once the decision is made to replace a measure, the question arises: Replace with what? Planning for a measure's replacement should be undertaken before the measure is into its death throes. If planning is undertaken early, an alternative measure developed, tested, and evaluated, the replacement can be an easy transition. Otherwise, the situation can lead to a crisis resulting in facile acceptance of an unsatisfactory alternative. Poor planning at this or any stage, for that matter, can lead to a second generation of sub-par measures.

If there is a moral to this story it is that what is done well early on in planning, developing, testing, and evaluating is likely to pay off later. We reap what we sow in terms of our performance measures.

# REFERENCES

1. Birkerts, S. 1994. *The Gutenberg elegies: the fate of reading in an electronic age.* New York: Fawcett Columbine.

2. Brennan, R. P. 1997. *Heisenberg probably slept here: The lives, times, and ideas of the great physicists of the 20th Century.* New York: John Wiley & Sons.

3. *CONQUEST 1.0, Overview: A Computerized Needs-oriented Quality Measurement Evaluation System.* 1996. President and Fellows of Harvard College (http://www.ahcpr.gov/qual/conqovr1.htm).

4. *CONQUEST 1.1, User's Guide.* 1996. Agency for Health Care Policy and Research.

5. Covey, S. 1989. *The habits of highly effective people.* New York: Simon & Schuster.

6. Davies, P. 1995. *Einstein's unfinished revolution.* New York: Simon & Schuster.

7. Donabedian, A. 1973. *Aspects of medical care administration.* Cambridge: Howard University Press.

8. *How to Score the SF-36 Health Survey.* 1994. Boston: Medical Outcomes Trust.

9. Kuttner, R. 1998. Must HMOs go bad. *New England Journal of Medicine.* 338(22): 1635–1639.

10. *Medicaid HEDIS as a Tool for Building a Quality Improvement System for Managed Care.* Conference and Handbook. Jointly sponsored by The American Public Welfare Association, The

Health Care Financing Administration, and The National Academy for State Health Policy in collaboration with The National Committee for Quality Assurance. March 14–15, 1996. Washington, D.C.

11. Moskowitz, D. 1994. *Ranking hospitals and physicians: The use and misuse of performance data. Volume 3.* Washington, D.C.: Faulkner & Gray.

12. National Committee for Quality Assurance (NCQA). *The State of Managed Care Quality.* 1997. Washington, D.C.

13. National Library of Health Indicators™, Joint Commission on Accreditation of Healthcare Organizations. 1997. Oakbrook Terrace, IL: p. 3.

14. Shah, I. 1972. *The exploits of the incomparable Nasrudin.* New York: Dutton, pp. 26–27.

# CHAPTER

# 2

# The Requirements for a Performance Measurement System

In order for a performance measurement system to be successful, it should be built or adopted by a group ready to design the system based on provider accountability. The first requirement is that the provider(s) be amenable to accepting the infringement of an external measurement system into their internal affairs (see Figure 2.1). It is, perhaps, because of this requirement that the true work toward the services of a performance measurement system comes about before a specific measurement system is even considered. It happens at a point in time when the leadership of a group of providers decides that the time is right to introduce the concepts of collective measurement of performance, collective and local evaluation of performance, and reporting observations and findings to audiences. In healthcare the goals of these audiences reflect the priorities of the times. In healthcare, it is not sufficient to do the right things but to do the right things in the most efficient, timely, and consumer-friendly manner.

An example of such an infringement occurred at the Kameda Medical Center, a 760-bed facility in Chiba Prefecture Japan—a two-hour express train ride from Tokyo, Japan. Kameda is the first and only hospital in Japan to be involved in the Maryland Hospital Association's Quality Indicator Project®, a research initiative that has developed a large comparative database on performance

*Continued*

19

*Continued*

indicators. Kameda joined the Project in the mid 1990s and continues to use most of its acute care performance indicators. Kameda has especially focused on four emergency department indicators (see Figure 2.1).

- Unscheduled returns to the ED within 72 hours

- Patients in the ED more than six hours

- Patients who leave the ED prior to completion of treatment

- Unscheduled admissions following an ambulatory procedure

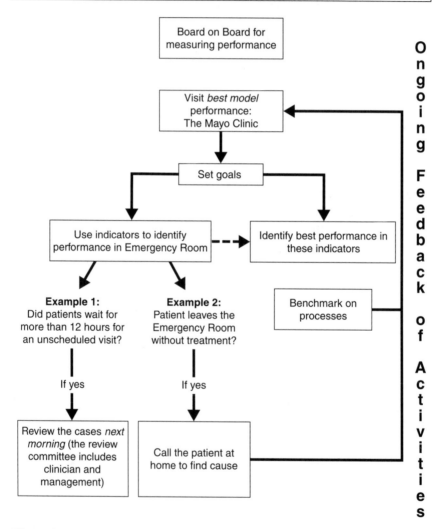

**Figure 2.1.** The vision of management as a prerequisite for a successful performance assessment strategy.

When resources are needed to build a performance measurement system, financial or in-kind support has been secured from such nontraditional audiences as business communities, potential patients, community organizations, educational and art foundations, and so on. Once providers agree to apply a performance system, they must begin to understand the profiles of need, demand, and community expectations. In healthcare, needs are defined primarily through changes in health status. Most commonly, those changes are designated as *diseases,* although needs can be nonpathological in nature. Needs can be further stratified into actual and anticipated needs. Actual needs are measured through the incidence or prevalence of disease conditions. Anticipated needs are based on the projections of the incidence and prevalence of disease, person-based historical trends, changes in vector, virulence, or environmental factors.

Epidemiological concepts as we have described them involve assessment of need as it pertains to people confined to a well-defined geographical area during a known period of time. Compared to need, the measurement of demand is slightly more probabilistic and is a function of provider, technological, and recipient expectations. Economic theory provides the basis to understand and quantify demand based on the request for products or services and based on the ability to induce demand. Inducing demand is, itself, a function of changing technology and provider behavior related to factors specific to the provider, ranging from personal economics (for example, target income theory) to the philosophy of the provision of services (for example, practice style).

Traditionally, medical models have been based on patient needs and how needs are addressed by professionals. The requests of patients or their families have played minor roles in models of medical care. Recently, there has been an increasing *democratization of knowledge* spurred on by enormous accessibility to various types of information through the electronic media, Internet, and satellite communications. These media forms have made *knowledge,* previously known only to professionals, available to a much wider audience. This democratization has resulted in increased demand on the part of consumers or their advocates for provider accountability for outcomes.

As on dimension of demand, it is not difficult to see how healthcare services for curative, palliative, or preventive reasons are influenced by the wants of patients. In women's health, there are numerous examples whereby patients' requests for a certain management modality significantly affect provider decisions. Common and expensive surgical procedures for women in every healthcare system in the world are hysterectomies and Cesarean sections. Both of these procedures can be influenced by patient preferences (for example, duration of labor) or quality of life (for example, uterine fibroids). Similar examples abound for many populations and conditions. Thus, the second step in the design or adoption of a performance measurement system is the establishment of baseline profiles of disease and population expectations regarding the management of their health status.

## UNDERSTANDING WHAT DIFFERENT AUDIENCES TAKE FOR GRANTED

When statistics are seen as almost irrelevant by clinicians to the assessment of their performance, we are faced with one of two strategies: eliminate systematic decision-making processes where statistical support is necessary in identifying the temporal profile of an event; or, demonstrate how statistics and systematic decision-making frameworks help evaluate services provided to patients and communities based on need or demand. Such a decision has to be made very early in the process of developing or evaluating a performance measurement system. There are a number of statistical tools that may, indeed, be of more value in understanding and interpreting rates and profiles than others. In this section we will discuss the concept behind statistical tests of significance and their relevance to the concept of performance measurement and continuous performance improvement.

## WHAT DO STATISTICAL TESTS ADDRESS?

The most common test of significance, known to practically all, is the P-test. As a test of significance, the idea behind a P-test is *to help the analyzer of the information discern those observations that are truly significantly, and almost unequivocally, different from the rest of the observations.* In that sense, the main purpose of a statistical test, if one considers a visual image of a normal curve, is to identify the events that significantly deviate from the mean of that distribution; those events will be outliers. Thus, statistical testing could be said to help the interpreter identify the outliers from the inliers. Statistical tests will also, in some instances, help identify the third group of observations which are fundamental to the understanding of data reporting later, namely, the *darn liers.*

Between this set of three categories, the outliers, inliers, and darn liers, how can statistical tests provide guidance and assist in performance improvement activities? The theoretical background of statistical tests of significance and their applications to performance improvement may not always be in concert.

If performance improvement for an individual over time, or a group of individuals (or a group of institutions) over time, is based on the belief that changing the level of performance (shifting the mean of distribution) necessitates a movement of the inliers, then focusing on the identification of outliers through statistical testing may be counterproductive. For example, it may be irrelevant or actually harmful to produce reports on performance indicators that identify trends or patterns based solely on a P-value that is *statistically* significant. It is, perhaps, more desirable to look at rates as a reflection of performance and not worry about the statistical significance of the difference between two numbers in making comparisons. The underlying logic is that if performance improvement is initiated only when there is statistical significance, such efforts will be undertaken only about 5 percent of the time. Thus, 95 percent of the observations (the inliers) will be left untouched and a shift in the mean of the distribution (and improvement in overall performance) may not be achieved. The immediate result of such a naïve strategy is the alienation of good performers. The long-term result is potentially hazardous: it is the destabilizing of a system without changing the environment. Sometimes, just tracking clinical performance can lead to significant improvement in indicator rates without any in-depth statistical analysis (see Figure 2.2).

Prince George's Hospital in Cheverly, Maryland, during the mid 1990s, wanted more information about returns to its intensive care unit. While its rates were in line with averages for this indicator across a large group of hospitals, the hospital quality improvement manager decided to develop a form that got behind the numbers in more detail. The form tracked complications for pacemakers, hemodynamic monitoring, thrombolytic therapy, key lab values, and ventilators (see Figure 2.2). This data gathering process led to a form that tracked maternal and fetal reasons for C-section deliveries. The form contained a graph with C-section rates matched by physician codes, comparing physician rates in the hospital to Maryland and national averages. In less than a year, the rate declined by 6 percentage points!

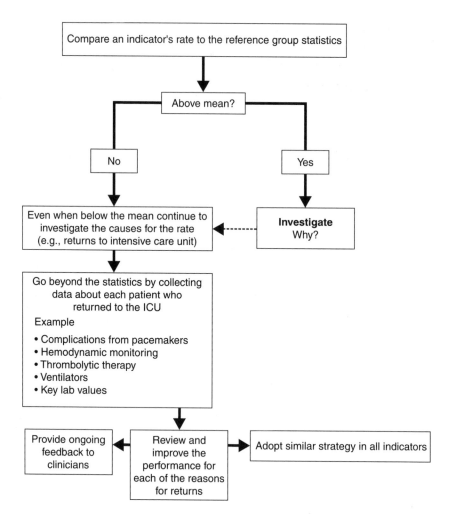

**Figure 2.2.** Epidemiological investigative methods used in indicator-based performance evaluation: The strategy of Prince George's Hospital Center in Maryland.

## THE STRUCTURE AND PROCESS OF DESIGNING A PERFORMANCE MEASUREMENT SYSTEM

But how do we structure a performance measurement system? How do we operationalize the expectations and goals that we set forth? Clearly, we need to have a structure and a series of processes to create a system where all the structures are dedicated to achieve a common goal.

First, there are structural characteristics that need to be in place during the design of a performance measurement system. These structural characteristics can be divided into

- Technical resources
- Expertise

Each of these structural characteristics will be discussed in order of importance. The structural characteristics regarding personnel are divided into what we will call the *project staff* as well as the external involvement of institutional leadership, community leadership, and the providers for whom the performance system is being designed.

# STRUCTURAL CHARACTERISTICS

### Project Staff

We recognize that the term *project staff* is not commonly used to designate the core expertise necessary for a performance measurement system. However, throughout this book we consider the performance measurement system as a dynamic process, which needs dedicated staff to not only carry it out but to treat it as an ongoing research project, always in need of fine-tuning. To manage the need and demand that are necessary, it is proposed that the project staff be comprised of the following:

1. An epidemiologist
2. A psychometrician/social scientist with a quantitative background
3. A clinician (M.D., D.O., R.N.)
4. A project manager
5. A database manager
6. A programmer
7. A communication expert

Throughout this book, special emphasis is placed upon the importance of epidemiology. We emphasize the portability of epidemiological concepts and methods in interpreting performance measures. The epidemiologist, at the core of the project staff, should preferrably be of *nontraditional vintage.* Specifically, the epidemiologist must have the flexibility to be able to extrapolate to the field of performance measurement, the methods of epidemiology. By extrapolation, the incidence of different levels of practice, within providers of care and recipients, can be measured through *traditional* epidemiological methods.

The epidemiologist is essential to the structure of the project staff because of the clinical background this person brings to the process of identifying critical aspects of measures and their construction. The psychometrician and clinicians provide immediate assistance to the epidemiologist. The psychometrician is primarily responsible for testing, evaluating, refining, and fine-tuning the measures once consensus has been achieved regarding their nature. By nature, the psychometrician is both an artist and scientist. The scientist systematically subjects each of the measures to the rigors of reliability and validity testing and examines the measure's factors that are used as indices of performance. The artist establishes an interactive, correlation-based model whereby the effects of different measures can be analyzed in concert with the overall performance measures. The psychometrician's artistic capabilities are essential since most of the performance measures are performers; they often can do no more than identify the potential for a certain aspect of care to be studied.

The clinicians can be viewed as *part-timers* at the beginning of the project. By *clinicians* we mean persons who have taken part or are active participants in the clinical management of patients. Physicians and nurses clearly qualify as clinicians, and a combination of these two job categories can be established depending on the availability of these professionals and the work demands derived from the nature of the measures themselves. The clinicians have two vital roles. These roles include providing a rationale, support, and guidance regarding the nature of the measures, especially their applicability to performance enhancement. These roles also include serving as spokespersons and leaders to audiences of clinicians or audiences responsive to clinicians.

Often there will be communication difficulties between the epidemiologist and the clinicians. This communication gap may result from different points of view or different *optics* used by each professional while looking at the same issue. The epidemiologist will look at measures applicable to groups of individuals; the clinicians will more readily accept measures that are applicable to individual patients. This dichotomy is expected, but must be rechanneled into a constructive and complimentary process. Indeed, not only the trees and the forest will be important in this process but also understanding the ecosystem within which those trees and forests grow. And it is at that point that the psychometrician will contribute significantly to the process by bringing the appropriate mind-set and approach to measuring aspects of that ecosystem, especially by placing the process within the context of social imperatives.

The database manager is responsible for translating the elements of the measures, as they are developed, into forms that can be electronically stored, manipulated, and will result in reports that can be distributed on a timely basis. The role of the database manager is important to the expansion of the project, both to new participants and to new measures. Without a solid ongoing team of programmers and database managers, the performance measurement system will not be able to systematically collect data. It will be unable to assess the completeness and reliability of data reporting. It will be unable to manipulate data and produce data sets and data reports made available to participants on a timely basis. Besides providing oversight to all these activities, the database manager will be responsible for supervising the programmers.

Finally, it is important to elaborate upon the issue of communication. Communication skills during and after the design of the measures will have an essential impact on the prompt acceptance of measures by the provider community. The way in which activities are described will affect their chances for acceptance and success. For example, knowing what different audiences take for granted, both in the amount of work involved in collecting the data and the possible and acceptable uses of those data toward the evaluation of performance, is a necessary skill each member of the project staff should have. Effective communication when the reports are produced, especially in the initial phases, is fundamental to the success of the project. We will discuss communication throughout this book as we discuss the limitations of performance measurement systems and how those limitations affect the interpretation of results. For now, suffice it to say that effective communication will serve a number of audiences, not the least of which is the internal audience, the members of the project staff.

It is easy to overlook important issues at this stage. For example, experts working on the design of a performance measurement system may start with common goals and aspirations and end up with different views about the process of getting there. During the process of developing measures—testing, gathering information, and communicating with diverse audiences—differences in perceptions may emerge among the professionals. We propose that the communications expert on this team, by design, should assume the role of facilitator, and serve as head of the office for both complaints and recommendations from each member of the project team. It is better to be safe than sorry when it comes to assuring that the project staff knows and understands the various details of the project design and participates directly in decisions.

## PROPOSED STEPS TOWARD A PERFORMANCE MEASUREMENT SYSTEM

A stepwise model of inquiry is proposed to facilitate addressing the fundamental questions toward a successful performance measurement system.

1. What do we need?
2. Why do we need it?
3. Do others know we need it?
4. How do we build it?
5. How do we choose indicators?
6. How do we compromise about indicators?
7. How about the environment?
8. Are we smarter?
9. A checklist?

## WHAT DO WE NEED?

To answer this question, each institution has to be faced with a competitive reality from its sister institutions in a geographical area. Based on human nature alone, change or the initiation of new initiatives will come only when the incentives are tangible and, in the case of healthcare, can be translated into the survival of an institution. "What do we need?" is a question that will be asked by those who have direct involvement in the functioning of the institution. Key groups that have that direct involvement include trustees and providers of services. Clearly, those two groups have very different backgrounds and interests regarding hospitals.

Trustees are community members that serve voluntarily on different boards and committees of the hospital. Their goal is to assure that the social institution is responding to the needs of the community and that the hospital fits within the larger web of services provided for the well-being of the community. Trustees have a natural mandate to oversee the quality, efficiency, and effectiveness of the services provided. The structure of a *trustee-based* community can be also found in medical care organizations other than hospitals.

Payers of care have a much narrower interest in keeping an eye on the performance of an institution. Payers are interested in assuring that their business liability is limited and uncompromised by the various practice styles of the providers. Payers of care are sometimes perceived as more interested in protocols, guidelines, and streamlining than in the practice of care and caring. However, payers are also interested in the effectiveness and production of health services. This twofold interest, namely in the appropriateness of the service and in the efficient production of the appropriate service, places the payers of care in a distinct category—a category of partnership. The question of "What do we need?" should be echoed across different audiences, including the payers.

The performance measurement system of the future (based on the experience of the past two decades in various healthcare systems) will demonstrate its vision by integrating various dimensions of performance. The performance measurement system of the future cannot be solely clinical in nature, but it has to include the dimensions of cost/charges, provision of services/management of patients, use of resources, and impact upon the recipients of care. This point is of enormous importance, because past experience has demonstrated that new answers to old questions remain within the context of the previous questions! For example, in most performance measurement systems developed in the 1980s and 1990s, "What is needed?" has almost always been answered by clinical algorithm demonstrating the goodness of care, a type of one-dimensional thinking that cannot survive the test of time.

Appropriate care is not solely what the physician or the clinician deems appropriate; it is not solely what the patient expects as appropriate; it is not solely what the administrators and the payers of care think is appropriate. Appropriate care is a synthesis of all these viewpoints. A successful decision-making model is based upon the operational construct of a performance measurement system that answers the question: "What do we need?" *we need an integrated decision-making system that incorporates the rendering of services and the appropriateness of those services, and considers the expectations of both providers and recipients by evaluating performance in the context of social acceptability and norms of quality.*

It is fundamental that the answer to "What do we need?" be explored thoroughly and thoughtfully by addressing it to different audiences. The project staff is responsible for the search for the answer. The leader of this staff has to promote a mind-set that the expertise necessary to integrate a decision-making system with management engineering has both clinical and societal dimensions. As such, the successful answer to the "What do we need?" question is a systemic one explored systematically.

The "What do we need?" question was addressed by Memorial Hospital in Colorado Springs when it created a *true continuum of care* to reduce its rate of unscheduled readmission. While Memorial had readmission rates lower than the mean of a large comparative group of hospitals, the hospital still felt there was room for improvement. An examination of the readmission data showed that the majority of readmissions involved patients with chronic heart failure (CHF) and chronic obstructive pulmonary disease (COPD). With the involvement of physicians, nurse clinical managers, and other staff, Memorial developed core care management models for each diagnosis (see Figure 2.3). These models were an outgrowth of the decision to conduct a close examination of a readmission indicator.

## WHY DO WE NEED IT?

This question gets at the *purpose* by addressing the values and mission of your organization. Are the values of your organization academic, economic, political, educational, philanthropic, or some combination of these? How will your measure help your organization meet certain objectives which flow from its values and its mission? Unless these questions are answered, organizations may find that they are wasting precious time and resources on something they do not need to know. On the other hand, the organizational introspection involved in addressing these questions may lead to an increased commitment of resources to the development of a performance measurement technology.

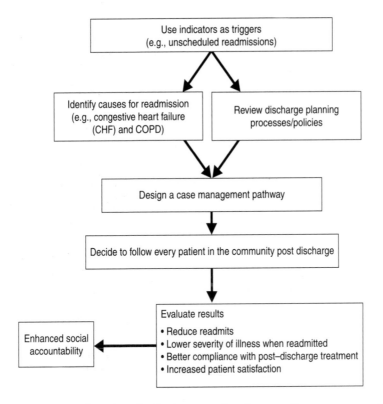

**Figure 2.3.**  Adopting a longitudinal approach to impact of care assessment: A study of readmissions. The Memorial Hospital in Colorado Springs experience.

The answer to this overriding question is less straightforward than it at first appears to be. We do not need the performance measurement system solely because providers, are interested in improving their performance. Although such a reason is laudable and an expression of professionalism, the impetus for the design of the system is often controversial. The basis for this controversy is inherent to any external auditing mechanism that would turn the designer against the auditor. In healthcare, auditors often do not share the same culture, background, training, and, in many ways, the same sacred circle as the healers. Indeed, often the auditors are nonclinicians who are given well-defined parameters within which they classify and reshape the art of medicine. It could be argued that external auditing does not really deal with the science of medicine, although there are differences in the understanding of that science among the practitioners. The variation that we observe in studies of geographic- or population-based studies is often a huge concern to auditors. This variation sometimes referred to as *small area variation analysis* is probably more a reflection of the application of the art of healing than it is of the healing's underlying biochemical sciences. Reducing this variation is, of course, one possible outcome of implementing a performance measurement system.

So why do we need a performance measurement system? Among the answers are

---

- We need it to demonstrate we are as good as our neighbor

- We need it because we believe that utilization and cost can be streamlined through more efficient production of services

- We need it to meet accreditation mandates

- We need it because there seems to be a noticeable departure from the norm in our ways of providing care

---

All four responses are valid, and all four deserve attention. Let us consider the last answer: We need it because of the observed differences in our performance vis-á-vis a norm. We first need to know how we defined or determined performance. Is there a systematic approach to the quantification of performance? More often than not the answer is *No*. It is, at best, the opinion people have formed about their performance from a one-time study they consider as representative. More commonly, it is the visceral grumbling of various leaders in an institution that confuse fact with fiction.

Second, we need to define a *norm*. What is a norm? What is a standard? Are those terms interchangeable? The answer is *No*. The terms are not interchangeable, and each one means a very different thing to different audiences. A norm is a construct derived from the pooling of prevalent behaviors. A norm will change as performance changes and will vary even when the standard is constant. The *gold standard,* as it is commonly referred to, is an expression of the scientific basis that will guide each performance practice. The gold standard for the management of pneumonia may be the use of a certain antimicrobial plus two days of hospitalization with IV therapy and standard imaging of the lungs, and so on. However, within that gold standard, the norms of practice may vary.

So why do we need a performance measurement system if performance is different from the norm? Being different means nothing in the absence of context. The norm, especially when derived from a small sample of external performers, can be inappropriate, full of caveats, or lagging behind innovative performance. Therefore, the perception that our difference is a bad difference and we need to look at how we can become similar to the norm is an insufficient reason to participate in the design and application of a performance measurement system. Considering the other two reasons given under this heading, we probably have additional justification for initiating a performance measurement system. If a system is needed to increase the efficiency of services, to streamline the various approaches, to manage the same issues, and to use the variable skills and resources in a responsible and cost-effective manner, a performance measurement system becomes an inherently necessary strategy to achieving those goals.

## HOW DO WE BUILD IT?

This question, perhaps, is the one that underlies most of the activities, or day-to-day operations, of a performance measurement system. Virtually all research and development activities must somehow deal with this question. Some of the topics that this question subsumes include the following: risk-adjustment, continuous versus dichotomous measures, data comparisons, statistical techniques, statistical reporting formats, data *purification,* reliability and validity, data standards, and confidentiality. We believe that problems that arise from this question can be minimized by adequately addressing the preceding questions in this list. Moreover, this question can completely paralyze an organization considering developing performance measures, either for internal use or for external commercial purposes. It is a question that involves a balancing act between scientific rigor and feasibility. The result is usually a pragmatic compromise that takes into account scientific demands, current operational practices, politics, and resources.

Once the initial discussions regarding the need for a performance measurement system have been conducted and an agreement has been reached between various groups to proceed with the design of the system, it is time to design a pathway for managing the process for the quantification of performance. Although the initial phase of agreeing on the importance and need for a performance system might seem to be a one-step process, there will always be questions regarding the true need for such a system. Therefore, part of the strategy in introducing the mechanics of the measurements is to continuously place these within the context of the need for such a system. Such is the strategy in politics "Don't give up! It is just when you are ready to give up (because you have been repeating your message time and time again) that people will finally get the message." Thus, persistence, a repetitive mantra, and good communication are extremely beneficial to the process.

# MANAGEMENT ISSUES

What is the pathway to managing the process of designing a performance measurement system? First, it is a team management issue. Indeed, there are numerous groups of people that need to be mobilized to contribute, and eventually achieve, the sense of ownership of the product. The most common groups of professionals who need to be involved in this phase are

- Physicians
- Nurses
- Nurse practitioners
- Hospital epidemiologist
- Academic epidemiologist
- Statisticians
- Quality improvement professionals
- Chief financial officers
- Hospital trustees
- Infection control professionals
- Medical records directors
- Information system managers
- Directors of planning
- Representatives of payers
- Representatives of business coalitions

- Professionals from home care

- Long-term care

- Psychiatric care

- Hospital public relations directors

Clearly, this list of audiences is long but incomplete. The completion of that list, at least theoretically, demands representation from the patients or of an ombudsman for the patients. When there are organizations that represent patients or potential patients stratified by age, gender, or condition, they should be considered and included in the discussions as necessary.

There is, of course, a major cautionary note associated with managing such large groups of people: the process may become so bureaucratic that most of the effort and time will be spent managing meetings, rather than managing issues. The success of this phase will depend on how the director or the leader of the project staff is able to communicate, manage, and direct the various activities getting the important issues exposed and discussed with all the above groups. It is desirable to have no more than two representatives of each category in various committees or task forces gathered to identify the issues. For example, considering the nature of most clinicians, putting two clinicians together is likely to result in at least two different opinions about performance dimensions that are being quantified. Although some diversity of opinion is desirable, large diversity of opinion may jeopardize reaching a decision regarding the aspect of performance to be measured.

The first task of this group is to come together, spend half a day listening to each other, and share opinions as to why a performance system is necessary, what are the drawbacks, what are the fears from each group's vantage point, and how they see the process evolving. During this first meeting, the team leader should be the project staff leader, who, always with the rest of the team, must keep a keen eye on identifying a natural leader among the group. It is expected that during this first half day a leader will emerge from this group who will have the intellectual, professional, personality, and moral requirements that the rest of the expert group will find necessary and appropriate throughout the process.

Once the natural leader of a performance measurement project is identified, the project team should approach him or her and start grooming that professional. The professional must be able to understand the field, and understand the efforts various groups are attempting in this arena. In addition, this individual must be provided with the necessary technical, clerical, and other assistance needed to reach out to the rest of the group members—to communicate the message frequently and forcefully. Thus, the identification of a leader from within a group of experts is a necessary first step that the project staff should complete before identifying aspects of performance to be quantified.

In designing a performance measurement system, there are a number of indices that will be proposed that are primarily clinical in nature. Indeed, it seems practically impossible for healthcare providers to refrain from focusing on clinical performance of individual providers or on the performance of an institution such as a hospital. In the hospital setting the most common types of measures are in-hospital mortality and hospital acquired infections. Unfortunately, both of these measures are insensitive, and their relationship with performance is highly questionable. For example, in-hospital mortality is often weakly related to the management of the patient, especially considering the potential of the patient for complications and, indeed, death.

Looking at in-hospital mortality can shed light upon performance in some situations, especially when there is a significantly atypical profile observed for a provider or a hospital. In recent history a number of mysteries have been solved by identifying an abnormal pattern of mortality and associating it with a single provider or site (for example, the *angel of death* in Ohio). However, such events are rare and do not qualify for inclusion in a generic performance system.

Nosocomial infections suffer from another shortcoming. Assuming that in the United States the average length of stay in a general acute care hospital varies between three and four days, it is noteworthy that the incubation period for certain organisms may often exceed the patient's length of stay. Misdiagnoses of hospital acquired infections occur not infrequently by missing the number of cases in which infection was acquired during hospitalization while the symptoms developed after the patient was discharged. Thus, those infections may be incorrectly classified as community acquired infections.

## THE CHOICE OF INDICATORS

The decision to focus performance measurement strategies on certain aspects of performance is a tricky but fundamental step in the process of developing measures. There has to be a set of guiding principles that can be put together by project staff and discussed with the group of professionals/experts who will provide the guidance as to which indicators are important. Those guiding principles should encompass not only issues of feasibility but also issues of philosophy (see Exhibit 2.1). For example, this group of experts may believe that most individual and group performance cannot be studied and evaluated in a vacuum. The contextual approach to understanding that is connoted by this philosophy may lead to strategies for integrating various aspects of service delivery and evaluation. In other cases, the philosophy might be primarily concerned with the measurement and evaluation of more traditional providers of care, primarily the physician. In those instances, the indices of performance will have a more clinical bent and should, therefore, be used in an appropriate context that does not detract from their validity.

No matter what the approach is, the principle remains the same: prior to the decision on the measures there must be a consensus about the purpose of the project. This is a logical recommendation, but it is one that is not always followed. At the start of the process of developing a performance measurement system, it is common to find that the experts, who are convened to provide guidance and steer the process, are prematurely presented with statistics and potential indicators. The impetus for such a hasty pace may be based on the belief that indicators are nothing more than statistics gathered from discharge databases and kept and maintained by hospitals or other healthcare organizations. This is a false perception.

*Indicators are often based on data collected for the purpose of routine patient management, but they have to extend beyond that purpose in order to be true performance measures.* In fact, most of the discharge data collected for administrative purposes have no affinity for clinical evaluation, nor do these measures have sufficient detail about the processes to provide clues about bottlenecks and inappropriate aspects of care. Thus, a performance measurement system based on indicators should specify, as part of its guiding principles, that those measures transcend existing sources of data, since their purpose is to uncover aspects of routine performance that will become key factors in understanding processes.

The day or two in which individuals are gathered to explore the types of indicators that will be pertinent to this performance measurement system can be an extremely constructive time for all involved. It should be expected that the experts have been selected because of their leadership, knowledge,

---

### Exhibit 2.1:

### Guiding Principles

1. Indicators don't measure quality, people do.

2. Indicators should be valid before being reliable.

3. Both validity and reliability are field-tested, not based on expert opinion.

4. Performance assessment is generic, but performance evaluation is local.

5. When people are willing to learn, even imperfect indicators can be useful.

---

and reputation. As such, they can be compared to musical prima donnas or to the first violinist in an orchestra. During the first gathering, it may become apparent that the role of the project director is to manage prima donnas, who are singing in a chorus, and first fiddlers, who are playing in an orchestra, interpreting the music or topic in their unique way. It is not an easy task; however, it is one that is manageable, if a plan of action is in place and each step during the discussion is anticipated and well orchestrated.

We said that the first meeting will be educational and constructive for each person involved. Indeed, it may be too optimistic to expect any suggestions or recommendations regarding indicators to crystallize during the first meeting. Rather, it will be a rewarding exercise to think of that meeting as a seminar or a forum whereby each professional and expert shares his or her knowledge and biases which will potentially clash with other biases around the table. A common understanding of the limits of acceptability may eventually emerge from this debate. We are careful not to require an absolute consensus, because it will probably not be achieved. Rather, what will be achieved is setting the rules of the game and setting the limits of acceptability of any approach regarding the indicator measurement system. The bottom line of this discussion is the following: The first day or the first session is a forum for all experts to get to know each other and understand each others' biases. Once the opportunity is provided to these experts to establish their territory and share their thoughts, they will be much more amenable to considering various proposals and to accepting compromises in the measures and their interpretation.

The next level in approaching the design of indicators is to identify the aspects of performance that are most amenable to both measurement and improvement. The amenability of those measures to improvement is fundamental. If the potential for improvement in practice, both at the individual or institutional level, is not well established, those indicators may not be a good choice (even when their data elements have already been collected or can be easily collected). For example, when looking at certain types of diseases and their present day state-of-the-art management, if the outcomes from the management of those conditions have not been affected by the process of providing care, then an indicator based on morbidity or mortality may not be a good choice.

If a measure is chosen as a clinical indicator but there are significant indications that clinical performance is a function of other *environmental* factors within the institution, then the choice of that indicator as a clinical indicator is ill-advised. Availability of certain imaging technologies, availability of anesthesia, and availability of special care unit beds all influence the practice style of providers and their choice of patient management. In those instances, to focus on aspects of patient management (without placing them within the context of other environmental factors) will be naïve and unjustifiably optimistic.

## THE ROLE OF PROJECT STAFF DURING THE IDENTIFICATION OF INDICATORS

A subsequent meeting is often necessary to discuss types of indicators. It is to be expected that a large number of ideas will be generated by each individual on the panel of experts as to viable or important indicators. The role of the project staff during this phase can be variable, but maintaining the role of *staff* as opposed to *expert* is advisable. Flip charts can be used to jot down all recommendations with the understanding that no decision will be made except to debate the proposed measures during this meeting. The discussion may result in more than one hundred ideas to be translated into potential indicators.

By the end of the day, sheets torn away from the flip chart easel and taped to the walls will cover all the walls of the meeting room. These pages will contain recommendations by the panel of experts to the project staff. Ideas are considered and evaluated by the project staff in terms of their relevance in developing new indicators. Later, the project staff will return to the panel of experts with indicators derived from those ideas.

It is really at this point that the performance measurement system mechanics start coming together. Those hundred or so indicators may eventually result in less than ten measures that are quantifiable, collectable, and amenable to performance improvement. Perhaps only 10 percent or so of all recommendations are translated into the actual measures for the first phase of this project. Of course, this does not mean that only ten out of the one hundred ideas end up being quantifiable.

Often, the redundancy of the ideas provided by the panel of experts and the significant overlap across indicators will be useful in identifying typologies of measures that will require synthesis. Once the project staff identifies those measures, an initial report needs to be produced regarding the rationale for the indicator and data sources. The quantification methods need to be identified, and epidemiological and clinical explanations have to be given as to how the findings from those measures can be used internally to understand and modify performance.

## THE BALANCING ACT WHEN DECIDING ON THE SET OF INDICATORS: THE COMPROMISE

It is rare that a consensus can be reached through the discussion of the pros and cons of each measure proposed by project staff. Perhaps not through consensus, but through a majority ruling, the set of indicators will be decided upon. It is important to decide who the final *owner* of this process will be. For example, when possible, the project director should make the final decision as to which indicators will be pilot tested.

If the proposed hierarchy of decision making is to be acceptable to a panel of experts, agreement regarding the purely advisory nature of the panel must have been secured prior to the discussions. These experts were invited to participate because of their knowledge and interest in the topic. The reward they receive from participation runs the spectrum from personal interest in the debates, to professional recognition, to more academic and clinical interest in participating in the research, to their potential authorship in peer review publications. All of these interests can be satisfied without the advisory group's veto power. It may be necessary to specify these functions and expectations from the beginning. Sometimes, as the process goes on and different experts get involved in different levels of the process, expectations may deviate from the initial job description.

No matter what angle one chooses to reach the decision about the set of measures to be pilot tested, the validity of the concept vs. the pursuit of validation of the measures will be important distinctions. The validity of the concept can be derived from expert opinion, literature review, or a combination of literature and ongoing research. It is during the process of debate and deliberation that the validity of the concept is established. Consensus or near consensus among the advisory panel and other group of experts is always based on the establishment of conceptually valid areas leading to the development of new indicators.

The validation of the concept and how it leads to the development of indicators is a totally different topic. It is a topic of epidemiology, and it is in the arena of performance improvement. Indeed, pilot testing the measures once they are mechanically ready (numerator, denominator, data, origins, exclusions, inclusions, understanding of temporality or incidence, understanding demographics and population characteristics, and so on) is a process whereby technically sound measures are tested for their usefulness in improving performance. A final decision on the choice of indicators should be based, a priori, on the perceived ability of those measures to improve performance. A number of requisites during that decision making become apparent.

The ability of the measures to improve performance is predicated upon the established track record of these measures in appropriately quantifying performance. If the performance measurement system is based on a continuum from measurement to evaluation to monitoring, then measuring or establishing the baseline of performance is the first task of those indicators. This is a phase of quantification that should carry no value judgment regarding appropriateness for measuring performance. The concept of quality does not enter in the discussion of this phase, although this phase is a necessary one toward reaching the borders that encompass quality.

Can a performance measure establish an epidemiological profile whereby the frequency of the happening is placed within an adequate time frame considering the group of people at risk for that event? In other words, can that performance measure become an index before becoming an indicator? In itself, this distinction is functionally and conceptually attractive. *The transformation of an index into an indicator happens when the index, after measuring the baseline of performance, is also used as a measure of the appropriateness of that performance.* As such, an index becomes an indicator when we go from quantification to qualification or evaluation. A true indicator is one that, in addition to measuring the event, can also shed some light in the direction of its goodness, desirability, and its adherence to accepted norms of practice. All these dimensions are an integral part of the larger and more elusive concept of quality. But the job of those measures does not end yet.

The third dimension in this continuum of measurement is monitoring. A certain capability should be built into performance indices, not only to enable their transformation from quantifying indices to qualifying indicators, but also to enable them to be measures that have meaning as part of a monitoring and surveillance system. It is an interesting concept, because in some ways it demonstrates the importance of focusing upon a surveillance methodology where the measurement system functions within an epidemiological logic.

## THE PUBLIC HEALTH LINK

It is possible to argue that the successful performance measurement system must have a major component of its methods, measurement, and interpretation dedicated to public health. This proposition is relatively revolutionary in the field of indicators which have historically been developed primarily for inpatient care. The historical background of performance can be related to the transition from subjective expert opinion to the management of care via a protocol. Unfortunately, the protocol has often been a synthesis of a few subjective statements by experts gathered around a table. Unless care protocols are based on the available literature and are frequently used to accommodate changes in science, the subjectivity component will remain high both among those who propose the protocols and those who apply them.

The way out of this circular discussion is to base the design and application of protocols upon the observations of a performance measurement system that attempts to relate the processes of care to the various levels of outcomes. Clearly, an immediate output of the process is what is observed in the patient between admission and discharge, a very short period of time for observing the relationship between the process and its consequences. Therefore, true outcomes measurement will be based on a performance measurement system that logically transcends the acute care venue (or institutional side of core in general which could include subacute care, rehab, and other) and follows the patient into the community. At that point, public health and medicine will be inextricably related, and the destiny of one will depend upon the fate of the other.

## THE TRIGGER AND TRAJECTORY MODEL

So far, this discussion stressed the functionality and sequence of events within a developing performance measurement system. The first issue is the mechanism of a *trigger* that will identify the need and opportunity to focus on a specific event or dimension of performance. The second issue is the *trajectory*. Following the patient's journey through the healthcare system into the community (in order to assess changes in health status) is necessary to evaluate the *goodness* and appropriateness of the process. The model we will discuss throughout the book is based on both concepts: trigger and trajectory.

**Development of Indicators.**    First, we will look at the development of indicators that are, in fact, primarily screening tools which will trigger further activity based on such characteristics as temporality, pattern, trend, or incidence versus prevalence of events. Those indicators are really triggering mechanisms to identify processes and evaluate their goodness. It is, however, incomplete as an approach to focus upon the goodness of performance solely from the angle of the application of the sciences of healing or caring. If that were true, the goodness of the process would have been solely an evaluation of conformance. By conformance, we mean the adherence to existing standards of practice knowledge accumulated through repetitive experience across time, region, and people, as well as a synthesis of subjective opinions of leading experts about the matter. The completeness will be achieved when the conformance to accepted norms or standards of practice has been supplemented by an impact analysis. The impact analysis is one whereby the process of that performance is juxtaposed and contrasted with the effect it has had on a number of audiences.

**Audiences.**    The first audience in this model is made of patients. The patients are both the recipients of the process as well as future inputs into the systems that will need the new processes. As such, patients become a very important fueling dimension in addition to being the direct recipients of these processes.

The second audience is made of providers. Provider satisfaction with compensation of their activities as well as the feedback they receive from their patients or communities will affect their personal growth—continuing their education, providing up-to-date services and technology to their communities and patients, and continuing to remain active within their brethern.

The third audience that will be impacted by the performance of the providers is the community at large, especially the component of that community involved with paying for the services. Interestingly enough, payers will pursue the same strategy that providers have but with a different mindset. Indeed, in order to standardize and make performance predictable, a revisiting of protocols, guidelines, or standard ways of practice will become increasingly requested by the payers from the providers. An actual example comes from a managed care situation where providers accept to play by the rules of the organization—agreeing to provide what the organization mandates and withholding types of services deemed unacceptable for one reason or another.

## WHO IS THE CHOSEN GROUP TO FIELD-TEST THE FIRST INDICATORS?

This question is one that involves both an understanding of resources available at institutions as well as the mind-set that will be conducive to the earnest testing of measures. Dealing with institutions or groups of people is very similar to dealing with entities from another culture. In fact, in healthcare any project like a performance measurement system will probably follow the steps and logic necessary to a worker going into international health. The following guiding principle should fare well with all parties involved in this process. The principle is: "the most important thing to learn about a culture is all the things people take for granted." The author of this saying is unknown, but the principle has been applied by many and successfully.

In the application of new measures through a performance measurement system that quantifies and evaluates performance, each group of individuals or institutions should be treated as culturally distinct. Institutions are known to have their own mission statement and values clearly elaborated on a piece of paper. However, it is practically impossible to find much variation in those value and mission statements across institutions. Therefore, value admission statements cannot be significantly useful when considering the best setting to pilot test indicators. Next are the providers. It could be said that hospital administrators and managers are predictable in their goals to maximize the livelihood of the institution. All the rules and behaviors seen in other business environments apply to hospitals and other health providing institutions. Therefore, the group that should test the indicators first is made of institutions with a previous track record in using quantitative research toward change and new policy.

## HOW DO WE TEST NEW INDICATORS?

A bad beginning makes a bad ending. (Euripides, 484–406 B.C.)

Field testing is an essential stage in the development of a set of performance measures. Generally, there is little justification for implementing a set of measures without testing them first. The development of valid performance measures and sets of measures depends on sound planning and evaluation; field testing is usually at the heart of this process.

Field tests can often answer many questions about the usefulness and interpretability of individual measures and may result in substantial changes to performance indicators before they are actually implemented. The extent of the field testing—number of participants, length, number of iterations—is a function of initial results, cost constraints, urgency of implementation, and the philosophy of the organization developing the measures. Thorough field testing encompasses at least five steps as shown in Figure 2.4.

Testing the indicators involves not only the collection of data as would be requested by the design of the measures, but also testing the usefulness of that data for improvement. In fact, the testing of indicators goes beyond

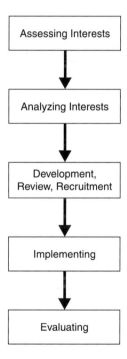

**Figure 2.4.**   Stages in field testing.

the traditional discussion of the reliability and validity of the indicators. In some ways the testing of reliability is relatively straightforward, involving the analysis of error and the analysis of its causes.

During the pilot testing phase, the reliability issue should be handled gingerly. It is expected that in most situations data, even when available, will not be identified or reported consistently across institutions. That alone should not deter the project from continuing. In general, the reliability of data collection and reporting will improve and will have an immediate effect upon the observed rates of those indicators.

There is a clear association between a well-organized institution and its image as a performer. However, an institution that is capable of identifying, collecting, and reporting information in a more complete manner will frequently have a *worse* rate, because its numerator will be more correctly reported frequently. Such artifactual effects have to be taken into consideration very early during indicator development. When underreporting is identified, the issues related to error of omission have to be addressed and their impact upon the comparability of the rate assessed. Therefore, it is primarily the reliability of indicators or more correctly the reliability of reporting that can be assessed during the pilot-testing phase of the project. That kind of testing, however, is not enough for many professionals who will be directly impacted by the implementation of a performance measurement system.

In addition to the reliability of performance measures, it is paramount to demonstrate the usefulness of those measures in their ability to capture true profiles of performance and help the providers of care improve as a consequence. Unfortunately, the pilot-testing period by most accounts is short. There is a hastiness in the field due to competition and external pressures to develop a product, pilot test it, and implement it as soon as possible. That approach can be counterproductive, dangerous, and basically inappropriate. It is not a luxury to take the necessary time for the development of performance measures and their testing.

There is a natural history of development just as there is a natural history for change in performance measurement, and both should be taken into consideration during the design of a performance measurement system. It is the goal of the system to induce change as well as maintain a level of performance that is optimal and acceptable. Those two goals cannot be achieved if one goal is sacrificed to the other. That is, if the natural history of development is shortened because of mere administrative operatives, a performance measurement system will be incapable of demonstrating any kind of impact upon performance.

Considerations of the natural history of development and change are under the domain and responsibility of two individuals involved in this process. The first is the director of the project who has the responsibility of directing the activities toward a functionally achievable system that will incorporate existing knowledge in the field, both clinical and administrative. The second individual is the leader who will emerge from the team of experts. The responsibilities of this individual are often overlooked, but fundamental. This individual will emerge during the early gathering of the advisory group and will have the unwritten responsibility of martialling efforts of the advisory team and experts from the field. This person will probably have regional if not national recognition as a result of solid accomplishments in the field. Eventually, the above activities will streamline the expectations from the field vis-á-vis the extent of validity and reliability that are achievable through the pilot-testing phase. Thus, the successful project will have the infrastructure to manage expectations through ongoing education in the field while simultaneously managing the design of the tools.

## PRETEST SURVEY

Field tests can be costly and resource intensive, and it is futile to undertake this process unless there is significant interest in the field for implementing the performance indicators which are being considered. Therefore, before field-testing new measures, it is often in the best interests of a performance measurement system to conduct a survey that assesses the interest of participants or potential participants. The survey (see example in Figure 2.5) should be concise yet comprehensive in content, readable, *user-friendly,* and clear; it should not ask for too much detail, but it should elicit informative responses. The survey should address a number of interests. Some examples of possible items to address are as follows:

---

- Performance measurement sets of interest (e.g., acute hospital, long-term care, or home care)

- Specific performance measures of interest (e.g., hospital acquired infection rates, wait times in the emergency department, or involuntary use of restraint)

*Continued*

Continued

- Form of data elements (aggregate vs. patient level)

- Interest in risk-adjustment or stratification of measures

- Strategy concerns such as expanding current performance measure sets, refining current measures, expanding the number of measures in current performance measure sets

Participants can sometimes suggest new performance measures that have escaped consideration by the organization developing the measures. Anecdotal information may be quite helpful to the measure's developers, especially at this early stage. Therefore, it is important to provide survey participants with the opportunity to respond to open-ended questions regarding performance measurement and measures.

Timing of the survey and the selection of a pool of knowledgeable respondents are critical elements for the survey's utility. Obviously, the survey should occur as close to the initiation of the field testing as is feasible; a long period of delay between the survey and the implementation of testing can lower the usefulness of the survey results in the fluid arena of healthcare. One can generally expect a response rate to the survey between 30 and 40 percent, even if follow-up reminders are sent out to all potential respondents. To assure an adequate pool of respondents, this reality must be acknowledged in planning the number of surveys to be sent.

## PRETEST SURVEY ANALYSIS

The survey data need to be analyzed to determine where the interests of potential participants in the performance measurement system lie. Since the survey is often comprised of a combination of checklists and open-ended questions, the analysis of data can be less than straightforward. In analyzing participant interests, both science and art play significant roles. The science lies in the structured analysis of the survey content; the art lies in the interpretation of that content. It is best to have more than one individual review the results of the survey since different individuals may see different things in reviewing the data.

The survey analysis should result in a report that is shared with members of the staff of the performance measurement system. The

## INDICATOR DEVELOPMENT SURVEY

**Return by:__/__/__Return to:** _____

**Directions: Please complete the information and survey contained below.**

**Survey Completed by:** _____

**ID Number:** _____

**Indicator Checklist:**

Please check the indicators that you would be interested in field-testing.

_____ inpatient mortality

_____ surgical site infections

_____ Cesarean deliveries

_____ emergency department wait times

_____ unscheduled readmissions

**Adding Indicators (Open-Ended):**

Please provide *specific* examples of other indicators you would like to field-test.

_____
_____
_____

**Additional Comments:**

_____
_____

**Figure 2.5.**     Sample of pre-field test questionnaire.

staff, then, become participants in the interpretive process and can contribute their own ideas about how to proceed based on the survey results. In the best of circumstances, there is substantial synergy in this process; in this case, the most promising performance measures are *thrown on the table,* as it were, as the group deliberates over their potential usefulness. This phase will end when a decision is made, either by consensus or fiat, as to which, if any, performance measures are to be tested in the field.

## IMPLEMENTING THE FIELD TEST

Once the decision is made to go ahead and begin development of a set of performance measures, planning the stages of individual measure development, securing expert review, and recruiting test sites are forefront issues. Usually, one person will be primarily responsible for the initial developmental work on the performance measures. It is cost-beneficial to the organization to base its performance measures on solid and comprehensive research. We have found that carefully written first drafts that are relatively complete in terms of definition result in *cleaner* and more efficient measure development.

While soliciting input at this stage from *experts* is extremely important, it too can be overdone. Involving too many individuals in the process—even if they are *experts*—can lead to excessive delays in development, overintense struggles about definitions, and needless conflict. If these factors are not controlled, the process can be undermined from the start. While zeal is necessary, overinvolvement by too many parties early in the process can be a stumbling block in development and can even lead to poor quality in the measures.

There is a right time to call in the *experts;* this time is usually when the issues are reasonably delineated and there is a well-developed outline or blueprint of the performance measures. Expert assistance in the development of performance measures is needed to ensure that the measures have face and content validity, reflect current realities in healthcare, and contain definitions and nomenclature which are in accord with generally accepted standards in the industry. Expert assistance can come from both in-house and external sources and can be representative of disciplines that are clinical, technical/informational, statistical, or administrative in nature.

Recruiting test sites involves an effective marketing and public information effort. The specifics of this effort—the marketing approaches and strategies—depend on the extent of participant interest and the size of the potential market that can be captured. The number of potential test sites can vary greatly depending on the type of performance measure, the location of the prospective sites (for example, northeastern United States, developing nation), and the types of facilities or services for which the measures are intended. If comparisons among facilities are seen as essential at this stage, then the more sites the better as long as costs and resources do not impinge. The willingness to participate in a field test and the extent of that participation are often very good indications of the future success in implementing the measures. By the same token, difficulties in recruiting field test sites usually signify potential problems in the future implementation of the performance measures.

At the time test sites are selected, information must be gathered that will allow the performance measurement system to assess the nature of those test sites, not only the data they submit. The new test sites should complete a registration sheet, such as the abbreviated form shown in Figure 2.6. This registration form will not only contain information about the test sites but will also furnish the contact person(s), essential addresses, phone numbers, e-mail addresses, and so on, that will be needed in follow-up.

In some respects, the implementation of field testing can be considered a milestone for the measure's developers. While there may be significant changes to the measure based on field test results—indeed, it may even be *shelved* permanently—the initiation of the field test implies that the measure meets a minimal standard of usefulness. Instructions to test sites must be *user-friendly* and thorough.

The field test should not only provide direct data from the performance measures but should also give participants an opportunity to express comments and opinions related to the measures and their implementation. It is useful to look at the influences of field site demographics on the performance measures and their feasibility of implementation. To do this, critical information about the field site (facility) must be obtained. Some examples are: utilization data, accreditation status, types of services available, environment (for example, urban, rural, suburban), and profit vs. nonprofit organization.

Note: Submission of this form is a requirement for participation in the field test. Please return this completed form by _____ to _____.

1. ID #: _____

2. Contact person: _____

3. Contact person's phone number: _____ _____
                                    Area   Number

4. Name of healthcare organization with which you are associated:

_____

5. In which state is your organization located?_____

6. Please indicate the nature of your organization (check only *one*):

   ❑   Home Care
   ❑   Acute Hospital
   ❑   Long-term Care
   ❑   Behavioral Health
   ❑   Other Please List: _____

7. Please indicate your organizational type (check only *one*):

   ❑   For-Profit
   ❑   Not-For-Profit
       Other:_____

**Figure 2.6.**   Example of registration form for field test sites.

# DATA SUBMISSION, COLLECTION, AND ANALYSIS

There are usually a small percentage of field test participants who will drop out of the study without submitting data. Other participants will submit incomplete or inaccurate data. This sort of *subject mortality* is useful information about the acceptability of the performance measures, their marketability, and their overall likelihood of success. However, one must make a conscientious effort to retain field test participants and see that all

1. Do you feel that this indicator's rates will be useful to your agency?
   Yes ❏          No ❏

2. If you were unable to report on one or more rates for this indicator, please indicate which rate(s) and explain why.

   _____

   _____

3. List any suggestions you have for improving this indicator.

   _____

   _____

4. Please document any specific problems you had with this indicator.

   _____

**Figure 2.7.**   Sample of post-field test questionnaire items.

data collected by participants are actually included in the evaluation to give the performance measure(s) a fair test.

The analysis of field test data often requires the same methods and technologies as the analysis of fully implemented measures. For example, the performance measurement system will likely need a data dictionary of all the elements of the performance measure.

The analysis is not complete without a posttest questionnaire. This questionnaire should address factors related to user satisfaction with the performance measure, detailed descriptions of difficulties, lists of suggestions for improving the measure, and any other information that will be useful in developing a valid indicator of performance. An example of such a survey is shown in Figure 2.7.

## THE ENVIRONMENT: EVALUATION OF RESULTS

The evaluation of the field test results is considered in the context of decisions revolving around three questions.

1. Is the measure ready for implementation?

2. If the measure is not ready for implementation, is additional testing warranted at this time?

3. If the measure is not ready for implementation and additional testing is not warranted at this time, what happens next?

The first question involves an extremely important judgment on the part of the organization developing the measure. While no measure is ever perfect, how much imperfection is permissible? There is no absolute answer to this question. Some things to look for are the measure's reliability or consistency of measurement, ease of data collection, perceived usefulness, and cost. There is also the question of how much can be gained by additional testing vs. the costs of more testing, both in terms of time and resources. This entails a cost-benefit analysis that must usually be undertaken and completed very soon after the initial field test data are available. In general, an organization cannot afford the luxury of a lengthy assessment of cost vs. benefits prior to making the decision of implementation vs. continued field testing, since field sites may lose interest in the interim. Therefore, there is considerable pressure to make this decision expeditiously. The decision is an especially difficult one if the data are ambiguous—not giving a clear indication as to the fitness of the measure for implementation. If this is the case, it may be better to err on the side of caution and continue to field-test the measure, since the costs of implementing a measure that is of little use can greatly outweigh any gains from speedy development.

The second question asks whether the organization feels that the results of the initial field test were positive enough to warrant further field-testing of the measures in the immediate or near future. Often, this is the case since some fine-tuning of the initial measures may be all that is needed to make them suitable for full implementation. Already, a considerable investment in the development of the measures has been made in terms of time, capital, and human intellectual resources. In all probability, some valuable information has been derived from the first field test, even if the measures are not yet ready for implementation.

Suspending the field test, or concluding that further testing is not warranted, at this time, can be ominous for the eventual success of the performance measures undergoing testing. The suspended testing scenario is most likely to occur when there is a lack of commitment to the measures on the part of the developing organization, possibly due to internal conflicting viewpoints about the usefulness and eventual market value of the measures. Basically, this stems from a lack of consensus about the utility of the measures even though a decision was made to initiate field testing.

There may be instances in which the field test results were so discouraging that a temporary suspension of testing seems warranted, even if there was strong consensus initially about the viability of the performance measures. Under this scenario, however, it seems more likely that instead of temporarily suspending the field test, a decision will be made to either completely redo the measures (go back to the drawing board) or drop their further development altogether. This decision is related to the third question: If the measure is not ready for implementation and additional testing is not warranted at this time, what happens next? In developing performance measures, it is occasionally wise to admit a failure, learn from it, and go on. *Continuing to devote time, capital, and intellectual resources to an endeavor that has not proved fruitful can drain the energy of an organization and keep it from moving on to more promising arenas.*

No matter what the outcome is, the field site participants deserve a report that informs them of the results of the field test. The report should be thorough without being tedious or stepping beyond what the data indicate. The appearance and organization of the report is extremely important, not only in communicating the results of the field test but in providing an example of the type of product that the performance measurement system is likely to have if the performance measure actually is implemented. This report can sell a measure or put a swift end to it no matter how valid or potentially useful it is. It is, therefore, important that the performance measurement system exert its best efforts in developing a field test report that will satisfy the needs of potential participants who will be considering whether or not the results justify the costs of implementation.

# INSTITUTIONAL AND PERFORMER PSYCHOANALYSIS

Performance measurement systems will achieve little if anything without considering the context in which they should be placed. Furthermore, that very context often needs to be structured and nurtured rather than just allowed to happen. It could be said that the success of a performance measurement is contingent upon the willingness of organizations and individuals to go through what we will call *psychoanalysis*.

The following anthropomorphic imagery can be borrowed from the field of clinical psychiatry to explain what we mean. Imagine we see a hospital, incarnate, lying on its back on a couch. Behind the couch is a researcher holding in his hands a report card or performance profile of that institution based on indicators that have been trended over time in a number of areas. The room is dark and there is a plethora of books and artifacts all over the area. The anthropomorphized hospital is staring at the ceiling and says to the researcher, "Now I know how I compare to others because of a pattern that I now accept to be true. However, I do not know why I am performing this way and what to do to change." At this point the researcher, without taking his eyes off the report card, replies, "I can help you but only if you are willing to be helped. You have to regard this as a collaborative effort. I am not here to judge you. I am here to help you understand your processes."

This jolly discussion is not in fact any different from the practical expectation of a performance measurement system. Indeed, that system will be just a triggering mechanism for further analysis, leading to a better understanding of the performance profile. The analogy goes even further. The researcher and his performance profiles will be of no use to the institution if that institution decides not to undertake introspective analysis and acknowledge that the established patterns are valid. The usual denial phase can very well apply to institutional behavior when threatening profiles are rejected as atypical, nonrepresentative, or artifactual due to deficiencies in a performance measurement system.

In order for the performance measurement system to work, participants must deal with the context within which it will function. The institution has to accept that the profile measuring system, although imperfect, can be improved by a joint working through of problems and issues. There has to be a kind of acceptability and good faith among all participants in a performance measurement system, a reasonable tolerance for some measurement error. It is, at the very least, relatively common to hear that unless the tools or approaches have been fully tested they should not be implemented. Such an approach can be self-serving; it is unrealistic given present-day imperatives for accountability.

All measurements in social science and medicine, in fact, all measurements period, will carry a margin of error. All science is imperfect, with imperfect measurement systems, with imperfect mind-sets of the interpreters, and with imperfect environments. Moreover, sociological and political imperatives can at any point in time influence the application or interpretation of performance measures and the sciences within which they reside. Interestingly enough, the last item in our analogy to psychoanalysis has relevance here about the nature of the couch upon which the institution or performer is lying. It could be said to be the couch of social accountability. The institution, given its social accountability requirements, is struggling to understand itself. In this process the researcher is using a set of established measures to facilitate this process of self-enlightenment or expansion of consciousness.

The successful and trustworthy researcher is the one who passes no judgment regarding the nature of a given institution's performance. In other words, the researcher using the performance measurement system is not trying to evaluate the performer but rather to help the performer understand its performance. A collaborative effort between the performer and the experts in performance measurement will, under favorable circumstances, lead to accountability to the communities that are being serviced.

## ARE WE SMARTER: CRANIAL vs. VISCERAL DECISION MAKING

When it comes to interpretation of information, healthcare providers seem to follow the predilections of clinicians. Those predilections often emphasize the *gut feeling* approach over approaches that are more systematic and cerebral. The *gut feeling* approach is one that assumes that subjective experiences are preeminent; the recommendation of external experts plays a relatively minor role in the final decision. The cornerstone of the difference between *gut feeling* and scientific approaches revolves around the importance of statistical information.

The topic of statistics, even elementary statistics, is a sore one to many healthcare providers. With some exceptions such as laboratory workers and those involved in the systematic manipulation of samples such as pathologists, providers seem to be reluctant to accept statistics as relevant to guiding and evaluating their performance.

A common misuse of visceral decision making versus more systematic or rational decision-making methods can be demonstrated by approaches to trend or pattern analysis. In trend assessment, there are basic recommendations as to how many points in time should be consecutively in the same direction in order to constitute a trend or a pattern. For example, eight or ten points in time regarding a certain aspect of performance or an output of that performance, when they are in the same direction, might justifiably constitute a trend. Unfortunately, such statistical recommendations are difficult to apply to healthcare realities. Indeed, eight points in time, irrespective of the direction in which they are going, often involve two years of data collection and reporting (considering a quarterly data collection process). In an environment where there is constant pressure toward accountability and demonstration of high performance, waiting two years to accumulate eight points in time may be an impossible proposition. Furthermore, it is likely that eight points in time will not be pointing in the same direction and thus will not constitute a trend or a pattern.

It is possible to minimize the problems associated with difficult data collection. One solution is collecting data on a more frequent basis. However, depending on the type of indicator and performance measure being considered, there might not be enough numerator events to constitute a valid and reliable rate for an indicator. For a variety of reasons, which run the spectrum from overvaluing an event to paucity of data, valid statistical or trend analysis is not always performed in healthcare. Many important decisions are made based on one, two, or three points in time! In such cases, it is truly the art of the management that is relied upon rather than the science underlying the evaluation of performance.

## A CHECKLIST FOR ASSESSING PERFORMANCE MEASUREMENT SYSTEMS

A performance measurement system must *perform.* If we accept that performance measurement systems can be assessed, we are then left with the prospect of developing a methodology for that assessment. The issues are: determining the specific items that are relevant under the three dimensions of assessment; deciding whether to weight these items in terms of importance, and, if so, deciding on a weighting system; and combining the dimensions of cost, access, quality, and user satisfaction for an overall assessment and recommendation.

Perhaps the most critical decision involves the relative importance of cost, quality, access, and user satisfaction in deciding upon a performance measurement system. Most organizations have an upper limit to what they can afford, so, in this sense, cost becomes an overriding issue. On the other hand, many organizations have lower limits for quality, access, and user satisfaction dimensions; at least a minimal level of *competence* in these dimensions is required of the performance measurement system.

Costs, both direct and indirect, are probably the most easy of the four dimensions to assess and compare. Direct costs are available from the performance measurement system, and, in many cases, it is possible to make a reasonably accurate estimate of indirect costs. Assessing quality, access, and user satisfaction is often difficult, because these dimensions are not so readily quantified. Some sort of rating system has to be devised that takes into account all the relevant items subsumed under these dimensions—for example, all of the items that are important to the prospective participant. Different raters may look at these dimensions from different vantage points so that it may be necessary to develop average ratings across raters. For those interested in pursuing this further, it may be useful to look at inter-rater reliability. One way of doing this is take the average correlation of ratings across raters. Low inter-rater indicates lack of agreement among raters and diminishes the confidence one can have in the results.

Figure 2.8 can be used as a tool to assess a performance measurement system. The tool has four domains: costs, quality, user access, and user satisfaction. Within these domains are various categories that allow potential users to provide more detailed ratings or assessments of the performance measurement system. For example, within *quality* there are twelve categories—five under *quantitative dimensions* and seven under *nonquantitative dimensions*.

Performance Measurement System

| Performance Attribute | ABC | XYZ |
|---|---|---|
| **Costs** | **Insert Actual or Estimated Costs** | |
| *Direct Costs:* | | |
| User Fees | | |
| Training Fees | | |
| User's Conferences/Seminars | | |
| Custom Reporting Charges | | |
| Other | | |
| *Indirect Costs:* | | |
| Computer Hardware | | |
| Computer Software | | |
| Internet Access Fees | | |
| Additional Staff | | |
| Travel | | |
| Other | | |
| Totals (Cost): | | |
| **Quality** | **Rate Systems from 1 to 5 where 1=extremely poor; 2=poor; 3=average; 4=good; and 5=extremely good** | |
| | ABC | XYZ |
| *Quantitative Dimensions:* | | |
| Statistical Reliability | | |
| Statistical Validity | | |
| Risk-Adjustment | | |
| Trending | | |
| Other | | |
| *Nonquantitative Dimensions:* | | |
| Relevance | | |
| Credibility | | |
| Comprehensiveness | | |
| Comparability | | |
| Clarity | | |
| Graphics | | |
| Peer Review Publications | | |
| Other | | |
| Average Rating (Quality): | | |
| **User Access** | **Rate Systems from 1 to 5 where 1=extremely poor; 2=poor; 3=average; 4=good; and 5=extremely good** | |
| Timeliness of Reports | | |
| Electronic Media Availability | | |
| Paper Availability | | |
| Responsiveness to User Needs | | |
| Presence of Help Desks or Other Related Support | | |
| Other | | |
| Average rating (Access): | | |
| **User Satisfaction** | **Rate Systems from 1 to 5 where 1=extremely poor; 2=poor; 3=average; 4=good; and 5=extremely good** | |
| Current Customer Ratings | | |
| Published User Survey Results | | |
| References | | |
| Personal Recommendations | | |
| Average Rating (User Satisfaction): | | |

**Figure 2.8.**   A tool for assessing performance measurement systems.

# CHAPTER

# 3

# Operational Dimensions of Performance Measurement

If you know a thing only qualitatively, you know it no more than vaguely. If you know it quantitatively—grasping some numerical measure that distinguishes it from an infinite number of other possibilities—you are beginning to know it deeply. You comprehend some of its beauty and you gain access to its power and the understanding it provides. Being afraid of quantification is tantamount to disenfranchising yourself, giving up on one of the most potent prospects for understanding and changing the world. (Carl Sagan, 1997)

## THE *SCIENCE* OF ORGANIZATIONAL PERFORMANCE MEASUREMENT

The science of individual performance measurement is relatively well developed for a number of reasons, including the urgent need for assessing individual differences during two world wars in this century. Conversely, *with the exception of financial performance and a few other relatively quantifiable measures of organizational output,* the science of organizational performance measurement is still relatively embryonic. We can think of four reasons why this is so. First, medicine, at least until recently, has focused more on the individual than it has on populations, leading to relatively greater advancements in the science of individual measurement than in the science of population, group, and organizational measurement. Second, as a culture, we are *individualistic;* the primacy of the individual over the group (population) leads to a greater emphasis on individual than group assessment. Third, by definition, the scientific studies of groups, populations, and organizations involve observations of more than one individual in various social arrangements; they are, therefore, inherently more complex than the study of one individual—or so it appears. And fourth, the *scientific study* of populations and organizations has less of a history than that of the study of individual differences—it simply got off to a later start, as it were.

### Opportunities and Concerns

Since our main interest is with the measurement of performance in organizations—more specifically, healthcare organizations—the developmental nature of this field, as a scientific discipline, poses some problems, but it also provides opportunities. While the field of performance measurement in healthcare lacks standard definitions, there is considerable agreement that performance involves *quality of care.* Experts have struggled for decades attempting to define this component of performance (Palmer, 1991). However, there is little evidence that one can generalize from the quality of care for one set of symptoms, diseases, or interventions to the quality of care for other symptoms, diseases, or interventions. There are hundreds of *performance measurement systems* which tap various domains of performance content, but there is little evidence in the literature to suggest that these systems are effective in measuring performance in any global sense. Few, if any, performance measures attempt to assess performance in an integrated and multidimensional manner, simultaneously accounting for quality of care and other factors related to performance.

There are other concerns in measuring organizational performance, which in healthcare frequently means measuring clinical outcomes. For example, in contrast with individual measurement, organizational performance measurement is typically comprised of essentially *one-item tests* which are often rates of adverse events (infections, mortality, readmissions). The dichotomous nature of these variables is cause for concern since the methods of analysis appropriate for continuous variables are not always appropriate for binary variables (Ash & Shwartz, 1994). In addition, there can be no item analysis for these measures since there is only one item on the *test.* Since reliability is related to the number of *test items,* unusual demands for consistency are placed on those collecting and reporting data for these organizational *one-item tests* of performance.

# DEFINING PERFORMANCE

While volumes have been written on performance measurement in medicine and other sciences, Avedis Donabedian (1980, 1982, 1985) is generally credited as the foremost contributor to current thinking about this ubiquitous concept in healthcare. Donabedian, however, has used the term *quality* rather than *performance* in explaining the basis of *structure, process,* and *outcome* in evaluating patient care. We will use the term *performance*, because it includes not only *quality* but such additional factors as cost of care, access to care, and patient satisfaction. While these factors are included within Donabedian's formulations of quality, we view the term *performance* as preferable to *quality* since the former term connotes assessing healthcare more as a science than as an art. In addition, *performance* is a term that has been used extensively in conceptual and measurement models in the physical and social sciences including engineering, psychology, and economics. It is these *applied* sciences which have most often labored over this term—both in its definition and measurement. Indeed, *performance* is a term with an *applied* connotation. It is also a term increasingly associated with the assessment of system functions and outcomes; we refer to the performance of systems more often than we refer to the quality of systems.

Performance can be defined in terms of its components. For our purposes, *high performance* is defined as the provision of cost-effective, high quality, and appropriately accessible health services that involve inputs and outcomes that satisfy the patient. *Low performance* is its opposite.

# A CONCEPTUAL AND MEASUREMENT MODEL

The scientific study of performance *requires* a model or paradigm. So does the design of a performance measurement system. We believe that a poor or incomplete model of performance is often better than no model at all—at least it can be improved. In fact, the terms *good* and *bad* are sometimes misleading in discussing a model. Models are either useful or they are not useful. At least in this sense, a useful model is a good model and a useless model a poor one. A useful model is well defined and its assumptions are explicit. The model serves as both a tool for understanding and as a vehicle for comparing performance within and between healthcare organizations—for example, as a measurement tool. Our conceptual model of performance is shown in Figure 3.1.

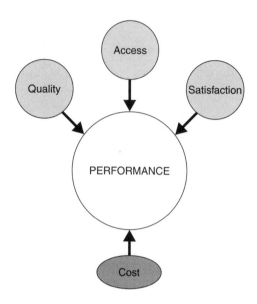

**Figure 3.1.**    A conceptual model of performance.

Our model is based on concepts borrowed from health services research, social psychology, and organizational psychology—especially field theory (Lewin, 1938), cognitive dissonance theory (Festinger, 1957), and expectancy theory (Vroom, 1964; Rotter, 1966; Green, 1992)—and adapting them to performance measurement in healthcare. According to our proposed model, performance is composed of four primary elements: *quality of care, cost of care, access to care,* and *satisfaction (patient, provider, and community).* Performance is positively related to quality of care, access to care, and satisfaction with care. If *value* is viewed as quality divided by cost of care, then performance can be seen as the product of value, access, and satisfaction. Mathematically, these relationships can be expressed in the following function

$$P = f(V) \cdot (A) \cdot (S)$$

where: $P$ = performance; $V$ = value; $A$ = access; and $S$ = satisfaction.

Since value $(V)$ is equal to quality divided by cost of care

$$P = f(Q/C) \cdot (A) \cdot (S)$$

where: $Q$ = quality; and $C$ = cost.

But *satisfaction* can be viewed as a function of several factors involving personal perceptions and expectancies. These factors are *perceived out-*

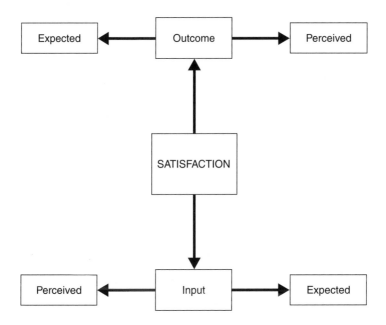

**Figure 3.2.** A model of satisfaction.

come of care $(O_p)$, expected outcome of care $(O_e)$, perceived input to care $(I_p)$ and expected input to care $(I_e)$ and are shown in Figure 3.2. These factors require some explanation.

***Perceived Outcome of Care*** *($O_p$).* This is the outcome of care as seen from the patient's, provider's, and community's point of view. Was the outcome *good, bad,* or *mediocre*—however that *outcome* is defined? The outcome, from the patient's, provider's, or community's vantage point (perceived outcome), can be changes in health status or functioning, symptom improvements, actual physiological changes as verified through clinical assessment, and so on. It can be a combination of any or all of these factors.

***Expected Outcome of Care*** *($O_e$).* This is the anticipated outcome of care prior to the medical encounter or intervention. Did the patient, provider, or community expect a *good, bad,* or *mediocre* outcome? The expected outcome and the factors that comprise that outcome are based on the vantage point of patients, providers, and communities. From the patient's point of view, did he expect that the knee surgery would allow him to play golf in two months? Did she expect that the medication prescribed by her primary care provider would relieve all her pain, most of her pain, half of her pain?

*Perceived Input to Care(I$_p$).*    This refers to the patient's subjective view of personal input into the medical intervention or encounter. Input, in this sense, is similar to both the *effort* expended by the patient and the *cost* to the patient. The *cost* is not the actual financial contribution of the patient but his subjective psychological contribution. A part of the patient's input can be the perceived financial burden; it is not a *dollars and cents* issue but a psychological one. In its totality, input refers to such things as the patient's pain, physical discomfort, inconvenience, anxiety, or any adverse factor associated with the patient's decision to seek medical treatment. *Perceived patient input is always during or after the fact or* post hoc; *it is the patient's perception during and after the medical encounter.*

*Expected Input to Care(I$_e$).*    This refers to the patient's *anticipated* personal input as a result of the medical encounter or intervention; that is, the expected input is the input *(costs or effort) anticipated by the patient prior to the medical encounter or intervention.* Once again, this anticipated input involves all the psychological and subjective factors associated with the decision to seek medical help.

In summary, perceived and expected patient outcomes and input are the factors that make up patient satisfaction by this model. But how are these factors combined? Satisfaction is a function of the ratio of perceived outcome *(O$_p$)* and expected outcome *(O$_e$)* or

$$S = f(O_p) / (O_e)$$

This model says that the more positive the perceived outcome in terms of the expected outcome, the higher the patient satisfaction. Simply stated, if the outcome was better than expected, the patient, provider, and community should be satisfied—all other things being equal. Conversely, if the outcome was worse than expected, the patient, provider, and community should be dissatisfied, again, all things being equal.

But there is more to this story. What about the patient's, provider's, and community's input—the sum total of the efforts, hardships, inconveniences, pain, and burdens that were part and parcel of the decision to undertake or render the medical treatment? Satisfaction should also be a function of the ratio of expected input *(I$_e$)* and *(I$_p$)*. The greater the expected input *relative to* the perceived input *(actual* input), the greater should be the satisfaction. In this case, at least in the patient's, provider's, or community's *mind,* the encounter wasn't as bad as anticipated—it wasn't as painful, inconvenient, disruptive, or burdensome. On the other hand, the less the expected input *relative to* the perceived input, the less should be the satisfaction. In this second case, the encounter was more of an ordeal than expected—the pain was worse than anticipated, the recovery period was longer than expected, the total resources consumed and ultimate burden to the provider and community were more than expected.

Satisfaction, then, can also be expressed as the following function:

$$S = f(I_e) / (I_p)$$

Combining formulas 4 and 5 yields

$$S = f(O_p) / (O_e) \times (I_e) / (I_p)$$

This model states that *satisfaction* is a function of the product of the ratios of

⇨ *perceived to expected outcome and*
⇨ *expected to perceived input*

In its complete form, performance can be expressed as the following function

$$P = f(Q/C) \cdot (A) \cdot (O_p/O_e) \cdot (I_e/I_p)$$

where, in case we've forgotten, $P$ = performance; $Q$ = quality; $C$ = cost; $A$ = access; $O_p$ = perceived outcome; $O_e$ = expected outcome; $I_e$ = expected input; and $I_p$ = perceived input.

## IMPLICATIONS OF THE MODEL

This model goes beyond the four-dimensional view of performance as a function of quality, cost, access, and satisfaction. *This model assumes that one unit increase (or decrease) in any component has the equivalent effect on performance of one unit increase (or decrease) in any other component. Essentially, quality of care, access to care, cost of care, and satisfaction are equally important as contributors to performance.* The mathematically expressed relationships are all *multiplicative* denoting an *interactive* or *synergistic* effect of the combination of these elements—unit or additive increases or decreases in two or more of these elements lead to *exponential* changes in performance. This model also assumes that every component varies on a scale with a minimum point of zero.[1] Negative values are not

---

[1]The model is most robust if the level of measurement is *interval* or *ratio*. It assumes at least ordinal level measurement.

allowed. While all the components of the model contribute uniquely to performance, the model does not assume that the components are independent. For instance, cost of care may be positively associated with quality of care (Burstin et al., 1993).

## Applicability and Variations

The model is applicable to the measurement of performance at macro or microlevels. For example, the model could be used to compare organizational performance for specific procedures (coronary artery bypass grafting, hip arthroplasty) or for specific diseases and symptoms. The model can also be applied to measure performance at global levels covering a wide range of procedures, interventions, diseases, conditions, and symptoms.

Variations that might improve the model, at least for some purposes, are certainly worth consideration. For example, one could posit an additive as opposed to multiplicative model—eliminating the synergistic or interactive notion of the components' effects on each other. Such an additive or linear model may have certain advantages when it comes to developing a measure of performance with desirable psychometric properties. Conceptually, however, we believe the multiplicative model is more useful than the additive model. One could also attach weights or coefficients to components of the model, corresponding to the degree to which the components are viewed as contributing to performance.

## Treating People vs. Treating Things

We view this model as a starting point for combining *objective* with patient-centered, subjective, and community factors in conceptualizing performance. This model is predicated on the notion that medical interventions involve treating patients and communities, as opposed to treating *things*—conditions, diseases, disabilities, or limitations. In still another sense, according to this model, the patient and community are seen as customers, and performance is related to the extent to which the need of the patient and community are met by the provider. It is not only the outcome as typically defined—the clinical result of the intervention—but also the *perceived outcome,* the outcome as seen through the patient's, community's, and provider's judgmental lenses, that is important according to this model. This subjective outcome is, in a sense, the *ultimate criterion.* But before we wander into a dangerous zone, we need to consider this notion further.

## Holding Providers Accountable for Subjective Outcomes

How can a provider of care be held accountable for the outcome as perceived by the patient, community, or the provider—the subjective as opposed to the objective outcome? We argue that satisfying the needs of the *public health community* and the patients is the ultimate goal of medical intervention. A well-informed provider, patient, and community can jointly develop reasonable expectations about the outcomes of patient care—expectations are in line with the empirical probabilities of the consequences of medical intervention. The provider's responsibility to educate himself, the patient, and the public health community is an integral part of the practice of medicine and certainly fundamental to our argument. This argument has found considerable substantiation in the recent literature. In the introductory article in a series on quality of care appearing in the *New England Journal of Medicine,* Blumenthal (1996) states that:

> . . . physicians owe it to themselves and their patients to master the substantive issues that underlie current discussions about the quality of care . . . physician's active engagement in research, teaching, and policy formulation concerning the quality of care will advance these activities and elevate the overall performance of our health care system.

## More Considerations

Detractors and *devil's advocates* may have one overriding criticism—that a *poor* clinical outcome can be excused if the consumer is satisfied— opening up this model to potential abuses by charlatans or incompetent medical practitioners. *Excusing* a poor clinical outcome is a clear misapplication of this model *since quality is as important in defining performance as satisfaction—it is just not more important.* By the same token, it is certainly possible to have a *good* clinical outcome and a *bad* result if the patient's and public's expectations are not fulfilled. This model addresses these issues since quality, access, and cost are coequals with satisfaction in defining performance.

Are there cases in which the model does not apply? We think the model has general applicability, but it needs to be modified for conceptualizing performance in some cases. For example, in treating small children or cognitively impaired individuals, the concept of *patient satisfaction* becomes problematic. If, however, we substitute *satisfaction of the public health community* in the satisfaction component of the model, then the model as proposed remains tenable.

## Summary of the Model

The study of performance measures and performance measurement systems requires both a definition and model of performance. We define performance in terms of its opposites—high and low. High performance is the provision of cost-effective, high quality, and appropriately accessible health services that involve inputs and outcomes that satisfy the patient, provider, and community. Low performance is its opposite. Our model of performance combines concepts from health services research, public health, and the social sciences. The components of the model include quality of care, cost of care, access to care, and satisfaction. The first three of these components are *objective;* the last, satisfaction, is *subjective.* The model is based on the notion that all of these components can be conceptualized and quantified. The model, since it has a mathematical basis, attempts to account for how all these components are quantifiably related to each other. To a large extent, the model is rational: it assumes that patients, providers, and communities can make valid assessments of the quality of care they receive or render and, if informed, can have reasonable expectations about the outcomes of that care.

We believe that while these components have been included in considerations of performance and its measurement, this effort is unique in its approach to linking the components. Our definition of satisfaction is based not on ratings of the elements of a medical encounter but on *patient, provider, and community perceptions* of outcomes and inputs vis-à-vis expectations. This is a formulation with origins in the social sciences as well as public health. While we still have no data to suggest that this approach is more valid than other approaches, we believe that its utility as a conceptual and measurement tool to understanding and measuring performance is worth investigating. It is worth considering as a starting point in designing performance measures and systems of performance measurement.

# PERFORMANCE MEASUREMENT AND CRITICAL MASS

## A Definition

*Critical mass* is a ubiquitous term in the organizational literature. However, we still need to define this term for the purposes of our discussion. *Critical mass* refers to the fact that a certain amount of some thing (patients, staff, resources) must be available before an effort, activity, project, enterprise, or organization is functional. If this *critical mass* is not reached, the activity or organization will be dysfunctional; it will not function properly.

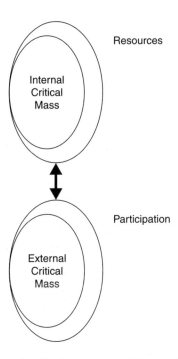

Resources

Participation

**Figure 3.3.** Two forms of critical mass essential to performance measurement systems.

## Impact of Critical Mass

There are two ways that this notion of *critical mass* comes into play when we discuss performance measurement. From the point of view of a performance measurement system, there must be a sufficient number of qualified staff to design, implement, market, and maintain performance indicators. The necessary capital, financial and intellectual, must also be available and in working order. This is the critical mass of the organization responsible for the performance measurement system. A second type of critical mass pertains to the number of participants in the performance measurement system—the *n* as it were of the performance measures. Without an adequate population, or an adequate sample from the population if you prefer, the critical mass is not reached and the performance data are extremely limited in their usefulness. In this case, the performance data can be said to be dysfunctional. As shown in Figure 3.3, a successful performance measurement system will meet the requirements of both notions of critical mass, internal and external.

# PERFORMANCE MEASUREMENT AND THE MOVING TARGET

## The Necessity of Change

If there is any constant in healthcare today, it is that healthcare is constantly changing. Change in healthcare is occurring in many ways including the way services are delivered, who delivers the services, where the services are delivered, how well the services are delivered, who pays for the services, and how the services are paid. In general, these aspects of healthcare relate to four concepts we have already discussed: quality, cost, access, and satisfaction. Performance measurement must somehow cope with this fluid environment if it is to be useful in tracking, comparing, and, ultimately, improving healthcare services and their delivery.

While all this change complicates performance measurement—especially when the rate of change is not constant but accelerated—performance measurement and change are partners in a marriage, however tumultuous. Without change, there is no point in tracking performance nor is there any reason to compare performers more than once. Indeed, the viability of performance measurement, as a discipline, depends on change.

## Impact of Revolutionary Change

Having acknowledged the absolute necessity of *change* for the development of the science of performance measurement, it must be said that extremely rapid or revolutionary change can diminish the reliability, usefulness, and validity of extant models of performance. New healthcare paradigms necessitate new performance measurement paradigms. We fear that the paradigm shifts occurring in healthcare are outpacing the enhancements that are taking place in performance measurement. Perhaps some examples will serve to illustrate this point.

Recent advances in genetics research appear ready to revolutionize medicine. These advances will not only influence how medicine is practiced in the next millennium (the processes of care) but will also impact outcomes (quality of life, health status). Performance measures designed specifically for this new paradigm in medicine are not widely available. Moreover, in addition to the processes of care, the structures in which health services are delivered are being radically altered. The emergence of integrated delivery systems and networks calls for new approaches to performance measurement. The provider of care that is being assessed is no longer a single facility (hospital, nursing home) but a network of providers

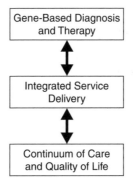

**Figure 3.4.**   Paradigm shifts that may impact performance measurement
at the start of the new millennium.

accountable to its eligible recipients or even a whole community. Is performance of such a system or network an additive function of the individual performance of each facility of which it is comprised or is performance, in this case, equal to something else than the sum of the parts? We suspect the latter, although there is precious little evidence one way or the other. Regrettably, there are few available measures to assess performance of integrated systems or networks, and there is a dearth of research on performance measurement issues related to this emerging and not well-understood environment. Figure 3.4 shows the three paradigm shifts that we believe are most likely to impact performance measurement at the start of the new millennium.

### Shifting Paradigms

If there is anything to be gleaned from all this it is that architects of performance measurement systems need to consider the effects of paradigm shifts in medicine when designing new measures or classes of measures. Measures and models of measurement based on twentieth-century paradigms are not likely to be useful or appropriate in the next millennium. While some clinical concerns are likely to be with us for the foreseeable future—nosocomial and surgical infections, complications following anesthesia—others are quickly fading and are best viewed as *sentinel.* Mortality is now so rare following many surgical procedures, where there was once a considerable mortality risk, that it is a useful indicator of performance only in special cases (certain open heart surgery procedures).

No one can predict the future with any certainty, but we believe there are likely to be significant paradigm changes in the next decade or two in medicine. There are only faint flickers on the horizon at this time. For example, performance measures which track and compare *outcomes resulting from gene-based therapy and testing* may replace or complement many current outcomes measures in the not-too-distant future. Conceiving and modeling *performance* as transcendent of specific medical interventions and as a function of the array of interventions undertaken throughout the *continuum of care* is another paradigm shift in performance measurement which may be felt in the near future. Unless performance measurement is able to be proactive—to respond to trends and changes before they become institutionalized—it will become a methodology illuminating the past rather than shedding light on the future.

# REFERENCES

1. Ash, A. S., and M. Shwartz. 1994. Evaluating the performance of risk-adjustment methods: dichotomous variables. In *Risk Adjustment for Measuring Health Care Outcomes*. Iezzoni, L., ed. Ann Arbor: Health Administration Press. 313–346.

2. Blumenthal, D. 1996. Quality of care—what is it. *New England Journal of Medicine*. 335(12) 891–894.

3. Burstin, H. R., et al. 1993. The effect of hospital financial characteristics on quality of care. *Journal of the American Medical Association*. 270(7): 845–849.

4. Donabedian, A. 1980. *Explorations in quality assessment and monitoring. Vol. 1. The definition of quality and approaches to its assessment.* Ann Arbor: Health Administration Press.

5. Donabedian, A. 1982. *Explorations in quality assessment and monitoring. Vol. 2. The criteria and standards of quality.* Ann Arbor: Health Administration Press.

6. Donabedian, A. 1985. *Explorations in quality assessment and monitoring. Vol. 3. The methods and findings of quality assessment and monitoring: an illustrated analysis.* Ann Arbor: Health Administration Press.

7. Festinger, L. 1957. *A theory of cognitive dissonance.* New York: Harper & Row.

8. Green, T. 1992. *Performance and motivation strategies for today's workforce: a guide to expectancy theory applications.* Greenwood Publishing Co.

9. Lewin, K. 1938. *The conceptual representation and the measurement of psychological forces.* Durham: Duke University Press.

10. McHorney, C. A. 1997. Generic health measurement: past accomplishments and a measurement paradigm for the 21st century. *Annals of Internal Medicine.* 127:743–750.

11. *Medicare Home Health Care Quality Assurance and Improvement Demonstration Outcome and Assessment Information Set.* 1997. Denver: Center for Health Policy Research.

12. Palmer, R. H. 1991. Considerations in defining quality of health care. In R. H. Palmer, A. Donabedian, and G. J. Povar, eds. *Striving for quality in health care: an inquiry into policy and practice.* Ann Arbor: Health Administration Press. 1–53.

13. Rotter, J. 1966. Generalized expectancies for internal versus external control of reinforcement. *Psychological Monographs.* 80(1): 1–28.

14. Sagan, C. 1997. *Billions and billions: thoughts on life and death at the brink of the millennium.* New York: Random House.

15. (SF-36). 1994. *Physical Therapy.* 74(6):521–527.

16. Stewart, A., and J. Ware. 1992. *Measuring functioning and well-being: The medical outcomes study approach.* Durham: Duke University Press.

17. Vroom, V. 1964. *Work and motivation.* New York: Wiley.

# CHAPTER

# 4

# Evaluating the Construct of a Performance Measurement System

A performance measurement system is a generic, systematic, and purposeful construct. The rationale for such a system is the same as that for other industries where a service is provided or a good is generated. To be acceptable, the measurement system has to pass certain tests of its construct and own performance. These considerations cut across social sciences, industrial models, and even pure sciences such as physics. In this chapter we visit these considerations in order to place them within the context of medicine and performance measurement. There is ample literature on the techniques and methods of evaluation, and our goal is to facilitate choice when evaluating a performance measurement system in healthcare.

## RELIABILITY

Reliability is the extent of *consistency* found in measurements of an event. Reliability is a function of *true* variation, total variation, and the extent to which *random* error is minimized. Reliability can frequently be improved by increasing the number of items (measures) in a scale or performance assessment instrument.

Normally, when something is measured repeatedly, there is some variation in the measurement even if the *true* value of that which is being measured remains constant. This lack of perfect reliability is due to chance or random errors in measurement. Another form of error is systematic or constant error. While constant error does not diminish the reliability of the measurement, it does negatively impact the validity.

Mathematically, reliability equals *true score* variance divided by *total variance*. This can be expressed as follows

$$r_{xx} = \frac{\sigma_t^2}{\sigma_x^2}$$

where: $r_{xx}$ = reliability; $\sigma_t^2$ = true score variance; and $\sigma_x^2$ = total variance.

Reliability or consistency of measurement is a necessary but not sufficient condition for validity. For example, if a person with a true weight of 150 lb steps on a scale that consistently understates a person's weight by 5 lb, that scale is still measuring reliably—*consistently* recording persons with a *true* weight of 150 lb as weighing 145 lb. However, the scale is not accurately recording the person's true weight—its recordings are invalid.

### Forms of Reliability

There are at least four types of reliability as shown in Figure 4.1: internal consistency, test-retest, interrater, and parallel forms. Internal consistency refers to the fact that the scores of items comprising a measure should correlate positively with each other. To measure internal consistency, Cronbach's Coefficient Alpha is often used (Cronbach, 1951). Test-retest reliability is one means of capturing random error, which can be defined as the random fluctuations in performance from one measurement time to the next. Test-retest reliability requires that the same measurements are taken at two different times and the results compared. Interrater reliability is the extent to which different raters agree on their quantitative assessments or judgments about an event. Finally, parallel forms reliability requires that two measures of the same attribute be developed and the results compared.

All forms of reliability assessment demand evidence of consistency or agreement. This implies that more than one measurement is taken of whatever it is that is being measured. Single item measures can provide no evidence of reliability unless a second measurement is undertaken and the results compared. Many current performance measures are, in fact, single item tests offering no evidence of reliability.

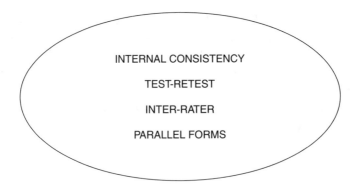

**Figure 4.1.**    Forms of reliability.

## *Reliability Necessary for Validity*

Acceptable reliability of each component of a performance model is essential if the measurement of performance is to be valid. In general, the more abstract the entity being measured, the more likely it is that random error will creep into the measurement and lower the reliability. Cost is less abstract and, in general, can be more directly measured than quality, access to care, and patient satisfaction. Its *subjectivity* is minimal, although not completely nonexistent. Hence, cost is likely to be measured more reliably than access, quality, or patient satisfaction. It is paramount that efforts be made to use indices of quality, access, and patient satisfaction that are also as reliable as that of cost if performance as conceptualized by our model is to be validly quantified. This is because the validity of a measure is directly related to the measure's reliability. For measures with a number of elements, such as our proposed model of performance involving four components, the theoretical maximum validity of performance would be a function of the reliability of each of the four component measures. Low reliability in any of the components would be extremely detrimental to the model's ability to accurately measure performance.

# VALIDITY

There are at least five types of validity which are relevant to the concept of performance measurement—face, content, construct, predictive, and concurrent validity. Predictive and concurrent validity are sometimes viewed as subtypes of construct validity, but they involve some important considerations that deserve separate attention. In fact, all five types of validity are not discrete entities but, in reality, highly related.

## Face Validity

Face validity is the least rigorous but most apparent form of validity. Sometimes face validity is more apparent than real. Face validity asks the question: Does a measure *appear to measure* what it says it does? If the answer is *yes,* then the measure is said to have face validity. Face validity is important in *selling* a measure or measurement system. Without it, it is unlikely that the measure or measurement system will ever see the light of day or get a fair test.

## Content Validity

Content validity concerns whether or not there is adequate sampling from the domain of dimensions, elements, items, or components which the measure should reflect. For example, if performance were viewed as strictly quality, strictly access, or strictly cost of care, its operationalization would not be complete—it would not have content validity. By adequately sampling from the domain of all components of a model (quality, access, cost, and patient satisfaction), content validity is assured. Content validity assumes that all domains of a model are sampled and that the sample is representative of the whole.

## Construct Validity

Considerable attention will be given to construct validity since some understanding of this sometimes difficult concept is essential in viewing *performance as we have conceived it.* One of the earliest references to construct validity appeared in an article by Cronbach and Meehl (1955), an article in which construct validity was essentially given its name. In attempting to define *construct validity,* these authors state:

> Construct validation is involved whenever a test is to be interpreted as a measure of some attribute or quality which is not "operationally defined" . . . Construct validity is not to be identified solely by particular investigative procedures but by the orientation of the investigator. (p. 282)

---

### No Single Index of Construct Validity Exists

For Cronbach and Meehl (1955), no single index is adequate evidence of construct validity. They suggest a diverse attack in attempting to establish the construct validity of a measure. Cronbach and Meehl list several types of evidence that are appropriate to support claims of construct validity. Among these are group differences, changes in performance, correlations, and internal structure. *Group differences* are considered as a type of evidence when the construct is postulated in such a way that individuals in different groups are conceived to possess different amounts of the characteristics or attributes involved. *Changes in performance* are important when stability or fluctuation in the measure (rate consistency or change) as a result of intervention or the passage of time are considered evidence in support of the claims as to the characteristics being measured. *Correlations* are considered important when two or more instruments are purported to measure similar constructs, or alternatively, distinctly different constructs. *Internal structure* is useful evidence for construct validity when the measure is considered to reflect unidimensional construct.

---

Performance and the various parts of which it is composed (quality, access, cost) can be viewed as constructs. A construct is an underlying and highly abstract *quality,* trait, or attribute of some person, place, organization, or other entity. It is not directly observable but inferred from observation. Using a personality attribute from the discipline of psychology as an example of a *construct,* the trait *authoritarian,* as a characteristic of personality, is inferred from certain types of behavior. This behavior involves a preference for strict obedience, enforcement of rules, and acquisition of power over others. The personality trait *authoritarian* is not a concrete characteristic that can be directly measured such as a person's height or systolic blood pressure. *Authoritarianism* is, however, a useful and heuristic construct that has been applied in a host of research studies dating back nearly 50 years (Adorno et al., 1950). Patient satisfaction can also be viewed as a construct. It can be inferred by a patient's behavior or the patient's response to a survey, but it is not directly observable. It is, in fact, an abstraction just as *authoritarianism* is an abstraction.

If the measurement model which was proposed is valid, then various indices of quality should be correlated with each other; they should demonstrate construct validity. This also holds true for the other aspects of performance: cost, access to care, and patient satisfaction. Quality of care should have a lower relationship with cost of care, access to care, and patient satisfaction than it does to other independent measures of quality.

This approach to construct validity is similar to that presented by Campbell and Fiske (1959) in a classic article which appeared in the *Psychological Bulletin.* These authors consider two types of construct validation: convergent and discriminant. Correlational evidence for the adequacy of a measure in terms of its *construct validity* requires demonstration of both convergent and discriminant validity. Convergent validation involves confirmation of a measurement by independent approaches. An example of convergence is a high correlation between independent measures of a trait, attribute, characteristic, outcome, or other construct (quality of healthcare). Discriminant validation refers to the fact that measures can be invalidated by correlating too highly with other measures from which they are intended to differ. Thus, access to care should not correlate too highly with quality of care if both are independent and valid constructs in their own right. Some recent research on severity-adjusted in-hospital mortality offers a good example of an attempt at convergent validation in healthcare research (Landon, Iezzoni, Ash, 1996; Iezzoni, Ash, Shwartz, 1996). This research concluded that there was often better agreement between severity-adjusted and unadjusted hospital mortality rates than between pairs of severity-adjusted mortality measures (Iezzoni, 1997). Different methods of measuring the same thing (severity-adjusted mortality) led to quite different results even though one might expect fairly close agreement; for example, there was a lack of convergence.

## Predictive Validity
Predictive validity involves an assessment of the extent to which measures are useful in predicting *future* events. Cholesterol levels in combination with blood pressure, blood glucose levels, smoking status, sex, and age are, in combination, reasonably good predictors of future adverse coronary events. In the education arena, Scholastic Aptitude Test scores are reasonably good predictors of success or failure in college.

## Concurrent Validity
Concurrent validity refers to the extent to which a measure correlates with or is related to some *present* event or phenomenon. Concurrent validity, like predictive and construct validity, is most often established by using correlation or regression methods of statistical analysis. High quality in a

medical setting should be correlated with high levels of patient satisfaction; conversely, poor quality should be associated with low patient satisfaction.

# RISK-ADJUSTMENT

## *Variability and How It Affects Comparisons*

Performance measurement is incomplete without taking into account the variability in the environment or in the recipients of healthcare services. If a healthcare organization is providing services to patients with an average severity of illness that is higher than other healthcare organizations in the comparison group, shouldn't this be taken into account in measuring its performance? Can the performance of a small rural hospital's understaffed emergency department be compared with that of a large teaching hospital's special trauma unit? To use an oft-repeated phrase, these comparisons are like *comparing apples and oranges.* They can be much improved if patient, organizational, and environmental factors are taken into consideration.

Risk-adjustment has been given considerable attention in the literature in recent years (Iezzoni, 1994; Goldfield & Boland, 1996; Aron et al., 1998). Risk-adjusted measures have more requirements than non–risk-adjusted measures. At a minimum, risk-adjusted measures require patient level outcomes, risk or severity data, an adequate population base, a method of linking risk or severity factors with patient outcomes, and a valid statistical methodology for adjusting outcomes. There appears to be growing pessimism about the current ability to improve comparisons of some clinical outcomes by risk-adjustment (Iezzoni, 1997). Certainly, research is inconclusive about the extent of overall improvement in performance measures by current risk-adjustment methodologies. There is still reason to believe that risk-adjustment will not disappear. Risk-adjusted measures are viewed as more credible than unadjusted measures by many practitioners and stakeholders in healthcare, even if it is often difficult to substantiate an empirical basis for this credibility.

## *An Example of Risk-Adjustment*

It may be useful to present an example of risk-adjustment using fictitious hospital mortality data. Such an example of risk-adjustment for coronary artery bypass graft surgery (CABG) is contained in Table 4.1. In this example, risk-adjustment is performed by using the American Society of Anesthesiologists (ASA) anesthesia risk classification system. Under this system, patients are rated on a scale ranging from 1 to 5 on the basis of risk factors.

**Table 4.1.**    Illustration of risk-adjustment of CABG mortality rates using ASA
classes to risk-adjust.*

| ASA class | Hospital X Observed # CABGs A | # Deaths B | Mortality rate C = B/A | Hospital X Expected # Deaths D = H·A | Mortality rate E = H | All Hospitals (n = 90) Observed # CABGs F | # Deaths G | Mortality rate H = G/F |
|---|---|---|---|---|---|---|---|---|
| 1 | 40 | 1 | 0.025 | 0.2 | 0.005 | 2000 | 10 | 0.005 |
| 2 | 300 | 6 | 0.020 | 4.0 | 0.013 | 6000 | 80 | 0.013 |
| 3 | 460 | 12 | 0.026 | 10.1 | 0.022 | 20000 | 440 | 0.022 |
| 4 | 200 | 10 | 0.050 | 6.7 | 0.033 | 18000 | 600 | 0.033 |
| 5 | 20 | 8 | 0.400 | 3.2 | 0.160 | 1000 | 160 | 0.160 |
| Totals | 1020 | *37* | 0.036 | *24.19* | 0.027 | 47000 | 1290 | *0.027* |

Risk Adjusted Mortality = (SUM Observed Deaths/SUM Expected Deaths) · (Hospital Wide
Mortality Rate) = (37/24.19) · .027 = 0.041

* The above data are purely fictitious and used for illustrative purposes only.

A rating of 1 indicates a healthy patient with no systemic disease undergoing elective surgery.[1] A rating of 5 indicates a patient who is in imminent danger of death. In this illustration, observed deaths are compared with expected deaths (a calculated figure based on the overall or total death rate by ASA class) to develop a risk-adjusted CABG mortality rate for Hospital X. Hospital X's risk-adjusted CABG mortality rate, .040 (or 4 deaths per 100 surgeries), is slightly higher than that hospital's observed rate, .034 (or 3.4 deaths per 100 surgeries). In addition, both the risk and non–risk-adjusted CABG mortality rates for Hospital X were higher than the *all hospital* mortality rate of .025 (2.5 deaths per 100 surgeries). The risk-adjustment, in this case, may have improved the ability to make accurate comparisons between Hospital X's CABG mortality rate and the *all-hospital* mortality rate.

This example of risk-adjustment was somewhat oversimplified to present the basics of the technique. Frequently, a number of variables are used as risk-adjusters. For example, in addition to ASA class, we could have introduced some demographic variables that may have influenced

[1] In *real life* it would be extremely unlikely that a patient assigned an ASA class of 1 (healthy with no systemic disease undergoing elective surgery) would undergo CABG surgery.

mortality risk in CABG surgery (age and sex of patient) or physiological factors (ejection fraction). Such factors are often included in logistic regressions or other forms of statistical analysis to improve comparisons through risk-adjustment.

## STANDARDIZATION

The components of a performance model may need to be *standardized* to ensure that the factors are actually weighted in the manner intended. This is because the actual variation, as measured by the variance or standard deviation of individual components of a model, is unlikely to be the same for all components. For basic mathematical reasons, components with the greatest variation are automatically weighted more heavily than components with less variation in models with no external weights (coefficients) supplied by the researcher.[2]

Standardization can be accomplished by performing *z-score* conversions on the data

$$Z = \frac{x - \bar{x}}{\sigma}$$

where: $Z$ = standard score; $x$ = raw score (unconverted data value); $\bar{x}$ = mean of population; and $\sigma$ = standard deviation of population.

## TYPES OF MEASUREMENT SCALES

Measuring scales are generally categorized into four types.

- Nominal
- Ordinal
- Interval
- Ratio

Most performance measurement models assume that their components are measured at the interval or ratio level. Measurement at the ordinal level, while not necessarily invalidating a model, places some severe restrictions on it.

---

[2] One alternative to the proposed model is a *weighted* model which contains components which are additive rather than multiplicative as is the case with the proposed model. The additive model is similar to a regression model, and interactive (synergistic) factors can be incorporated.

*Nominal scales* allow placement into categories. An example would be demographic data (sex, race, and age) and some types of outcome data such as patient mortality—the patient either survived or expired. Few statistical tests of association can be performed on this type of scale. However, one appropriate test is the chi-square test of statistical significance.

*Ordinal scales* allow for the rank ordering of data. The mode and median are acceptable measures of central tendency for ordinal scales. Percentiles may be used as a measure of dispersion, and rank-order (rho) correlation is an appropriate test of association.

*Interval scales,* probably the most common type of scale in the social and biological sciences, allow three measures of central tendency: mean, mode, and median. Measures of dispersion, which are appropriate, include the variance and its square root, the standard deviation. Various correlational and regression methods are appropriate for estimating association. Interval scales do not have an absolute zero point.

*Ratio scales* have an absolute zero. Celsius and Fahrenheit scales are good examples. Measures of central tendency include mode, mean, median, harmonic, and geometric mean. Percent variation is an appropriate dispersion statistic and numerous tests of association can be used without violating the assumptions of this type of scale, including correlation and regression techniques.

In general, physical measurements can be made at the level of ratio scales, since they usually have an absolute zero. Measurements on hypothetical constructs or on psychological variables generally are made on the level of interval scales. For example, it would be difficult to consider an individual as having an IQ of zero, a requirement for a ratio scale. Many physiological measurements have an absolute zero point.

The types of measurement scales are important to remember, and it is also important to be able to categorize our measurement tool in terms of the appropriate measurement scale. Researchers may unwittingly try to combine nominal data and end up with results that are meaningless. The numbers on the backs of shirts of football players are nominal data—they are only meaningful in helping to identify players (a type of categorization). Adding or combining these numbers makes no sense. While this is obvious, it may not be so obvious to researchers attempting to combine more esoteric but essentially nominal data.

# THE NORMAL DISTRIBUTION

The *normal distribution* is probably best known as the bell-shaped curve, symmetrical and extending in both directions infinitely far. This curve has certain mathematical properties that are defined and discussed at length in almost any intermediate level statistics book. This is not a text on statistical methods, and we will not discuss these properties at length here. However, we think it important to state that while this curve may be *normal,* there is no particular reason to expect that all populations sampled will display this distribution. What we can expect is that the sample distribution of population means tends to be normal even if the universe of data points is not normally distributed. This is the *central limit theorem:*

> . . . the sampling distribution of the means of random samples will be approximately normal in form regardless of the form of the distribution in the population, provided the sample size is sufficiently large and provided that the population variance is finite. (Winer, 1971)

Many naturally occurring phenomena are nearly normally distributed, however. They include systolic and diastolic blood pressures of adults, heights and weights of adults, and intelligence quotient (IQ) scores. Indeed the normal curve is a good approximation for a host of phenomena.

Some performance indicators bear a close approximation to normal distributions. An example of this is Cesarean section rates taken from a large sample of hospitals. Such a distribution may look something like the hypothetical distribution contained in Figure 4.2.

# SKEWED DISTRIBUTIONS

Unlike the example for Cesarean delivery rates, our experience is that most performance indicators in healthcare have distributions that do not approximate the normal distribution. This fact presents some problems when methods of reporting and analysis assume at least an approximation of the normal distribution. For example, the standard deviation is often used as a measure of variation in performance indicator rates. The value of this statistic is questionable when the distribution is a highly skewed or Poisson distribution. The hypothetical example in Figure 4.3 illustrates a highly skewed distribution—the type of distribution that one might find in reporting surgical infection rates.

The mean of the distribution is 2.2 infections per 100 patients. The standard deviation of this distribution is 2.7. Just one standard deviation below

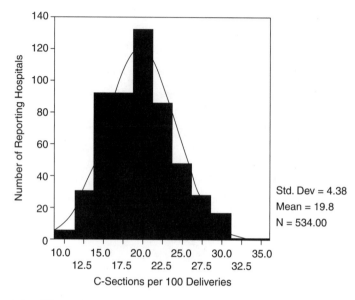

**Figure 4.2.**  Illustration of distribution of Cesarean delivery rates.

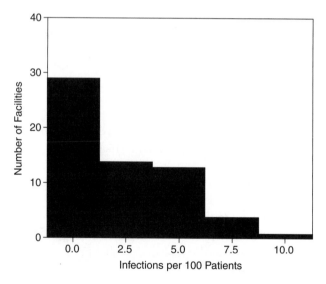

**Figure 4.3.**  Surgical infection rates per 100 patients by number
of facilities reporting.

the mean translates to a negative number, which is impossible! The median of this distribution is 2.0 and is below the mean of 2.2. This is another characteristic of skewed distributions: the mean is higher than the median.

The situation depicted here is commonplace in performance measures of this type: a positively skewed distribution (the tail extends to the right). Interpretation of data at the facility level can often be problematic under this type of scenario. For example, what does it mean to have a facility rate of 1.5 infections per 100 patients, which is considerably below the mean but higher than a substantial percentage of those reporting? In fact, nearly 30 percent of the facilities in the illustration had a reported infection rate of 0. Is this realistic? Does it reflect accurate reporting? These questions defy general answers; they can only be addressed on a case-by-case basis.

One way of ameliorating the effects of such skewed data is to average observations over several reporting periods. This allows individual reporting facilities to arrive at a better overall comparison of their performance with that of their peers than is available on the basis of one reporting period. The disadvantage of this approach is the lack of timeliness and relevance of the information as conditions and circumstances change for performance assessment. Accumulating a year's worth of data instead of, let's say, one quarter's worth–available, perhaps, as late as 15 months after the start of the reporting period–may or may not prove to be beneficial to those using the data. There is really a trade-off between timing and the ability to interpret the data. Decisions as to which are most important are beyond the purview of the performance measurement system; they should be handled at the provider's level.

A second way of minimizing the problems inherent in skewed distributions of performance rates is to use the data to set levels or thresholds for acceptable performance. Usually these thresholds are set at some extreme value. For example, facilities that are consistently above the 90th or 95th percentile[3] in such distributions may want to take a closer look at their performance to determine if structures or processes need to be revamped or modified. Thus, despite some inherent problems in interpreting skewed data, they can be used effectively by healthcare facilities with rates consistently near or above thresholds of acceptable performance. Skewed data, especially if highly skewed, are less helpful to healthcare providers with consistently average performance scores (or slightly deviating from average) that wish to use the data to measure performance improvement.

---

[3] The percentage of observations in a distribution that is at or below a given rate or score.

# SENTINEL INDICATORS

According to *Webster's Revised Unabridged Dictionary, sentinel* refers to *one who watches or guards; specifically, a soldier set to guard an army, camp, or other place, from surprise, to observe the approach of danger, and give notice of it; a sentry.* It is the part of the definition which deals with observing and giving notice to the approach of danger that is most relevant for our purposes. *Sentinel* is commonly used to refer to performance indicators that measure rare and unexpected events resulting in serious physical or psychological harm or at least the risk of serious injury. There are numerous studies on sentinel or adverse events occurring in healthcare settings, especially in hospitals (Brennan, 1991; Leape, 1991; Garcia-Martin et al., 1997).

Sentinel indicators represent an extreme of the quantitative problems inherent with skewed distributions. Distributions of events or rates for sentinel indicators are extremely skewed. Examples of rare and unexpected, adverse events that have been used as sentinel indicators include inpatient suicide (assisted or nonassisted), inpatient homicide, certain other forms of purposeful self-injurious behavior or behavior injurious to others, mortality or other adverse outcomes not usually associated with certain patient conditions or treatments, and egregious errors in medication administration or other forms of treatment that result in serious injury.

A hypothetical example of a sentinel indicator is depicted in Figure 4.4. A rare injurious event, *physical assault in psychiatric facilities* is reduced to its rate of occurrence per 100 patient days and plotted against the number of reporting facilities. The mean rate of physical assaults per 100 patient days across 106 reporting facilities is 0.1. The standard deviation is 0.53. The mode of this distribution is 0; a total of 100 of the 106 facilities report no physical assaults.

From a psychometric point of view, sentinel indicators are virtually impossible to assess. Standard measures of reliability and validity just do not seem to apply to sentinel indicators. How do you use performance measures that capture something so fleeting—so ephemeral as sentinel events? We know of no completely satisfactory answer to this question. It is safe to say, however, that sentinel indicators are better used in *monitoring* events than they are for measuring performance. They cannot be discounted, because the events they capture are too

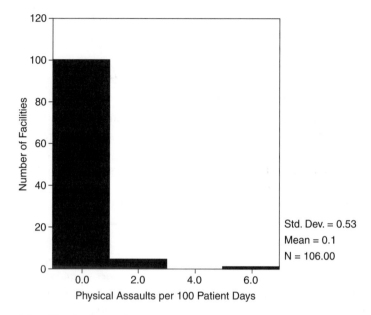

**Figure 4.4.** Physical assault rates per 100 psychiatric patients by number of facilities.

critical and injurious to patient health and well-being. Sentinel indicators may reveal some underlying flaw in structure or process in a healthcare organization, or, alternatively, they may reflect nothing more than a random happening. That interpretation has to be made by the provider, its accreditation and regulatory agencies, and, occasionally, by legal agencies and the courts.

## DATA TRANSFORMATIONS

Two general types of data transformations can occur: the transformation of numerical data to nominal data and the transformation of numerical data into other numerical data in a one-to-one continuous fashion. The former has been termed *discrete transformation* and the latter, *continuous transformation* (Bailey, 1971).

The distortion inherent in skewed distributions can sometimes be greatly diminished by logarithmic transformation, a form of continuous transformation. Logarithmic transformation is, however, not to be taken lightly. This and other data transformations may be permissible under one set of conditions and completely impermissible under other conditions.

## BINARY vs. CONTINUOUS VARIABLES AS PERFORMANCE MEASURES

Binary or dichotomous variables take on a value of *1* or *0*. Some examples from hospital performance measurement are inpatient mortality and read-missions. It is clear that a patient is either discharged alive or dead or is readmitted or is not readmitted in a given time frame. There can be no intermediate values.

> With binary (dichotomous variables), the formula for the *variance* of the distribution of numerical values (binomial distribution) is: $\sigma^2 = p\,(1-p)/n$. *Where:* $\sigma^2$ = *variance,* p = *probability of event* x *(mean), and* n = *number of cases. Remember that* p = *(occurrences/(occurrences + nonoccurrences))* *or, alternatively,* p = *(occurrences/events). The standard deviation of the distribution is the square root of the variance* ($\sigma^2$).

To describe a distribution of binary variables, it is only necessary to have two data elements: the numerator and the denominator. Typically, the numerator contains the number of events that occurred (deaths), and the denominator contains the number of cases (the number of occurrences and the number of nonoccurrences of the event). For binary variables, *aggregate* data are thus sufficient to describe the distribution of data values.

For continuous variables (variables with more than two values), either patient-level data or case counts are required for all possible data values. In most cases, patient-level data (one record per patient) are submitted from providers of care to the performance measurement system when performance outcomes are measured on a continuum with more than two data values.

## PUBLIC ACCOUNTABILITY AND QUALITY IMPROVEMENT: DIFFERENT OBJECTIVES OF PERFORMANCE MEASUREMENT

The design of performance measures depends on which of two objectives the measures are intended to address: (1) to provide information useful for

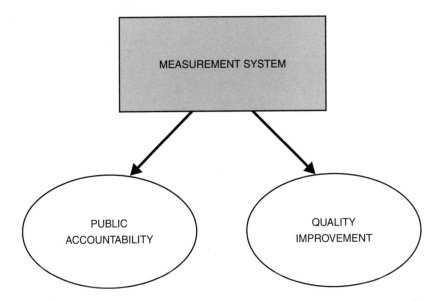

**Figure 4.5.**  Objectives of measurement.

quality improvement or (2) to satisfy concerns raised by the public related to accountability. These objectives are shown in Figure 4.5. Depending on the major objective, the design of the performance measures may be substantially different. Measures built primarily for improving performance—usually by identifying processes that need to be improved—will often not need to be risk-adjusted. These measures will be specifically applicable to the institutions and settings in which quality improvement is of immediate concern. They may not have general applicability over a wide range of settings and institutions. On the other hand, measures designed to meet demands for accountability must be useful in making comparisons across institutions. They will almost certainly have a mechanism for risk-adjustment (or at least stratification) in an attempt to attain a level playing field to conduct institutional comparisons. These measures will likely involve a high need for scientific rigor. They will generally be outcome-based and must demonstrate reliability and validity in the populations in which they are being used. Usually, they must undergo extensive development and field testing before they are introduced.

Confusion about these very different objectives of the performance measurement system can lead to inappropriate performance measures and unnecessary resource outlays in development. For example, if one is only interested in improving internal processes, then why spend time and resources in developing sophisticated risk-adjustment measures? Conversely, if one's interest is in developing measures that will be useful for comparing one institution with another in terms of clinical outcomes, why concern oneself with the idiosyncratic processes of care among institutions.

Some measurement systems may attempt to develop performance measures that meet both the objectives of public accountability and internal quality improvement *at the same time.* These measures must be acceptable to a wide range of individuals from various disciplines: statisticians and psychometricians, clinicians, quality assurance directors, administrators, payers, regulators, and leaders of employee and consumer groups. Attempting to be all things to all people can, indeed, be a daunting task, but it is one faced by many performance measurement systems concerned with both public accountability and quality improvement goals.

## SUMMARY OF MEASUREMENT ISSUES

Reliability is the consistency of measurement of an event; it comes to us in various forms—test-retest, alternate forms, and internal consistency. From a psychometric viewpoint, the *sine qua non* of performance measurement is reliability. Without reliability of measurement, there can be no validity of measurement. With multiple measures and or multiple components in a mathematical expression, minor variations in reliability in one or more of the components can have major consequences. Reliability, while necessary for validity, does not assure validity. One can measure something consistently while measuring it incorrectly.

Validity is the extent to which something measures what it says it measures. Like reliability, it also has various forms. Among these are face, content, construct, and predictive validity. The current state of affairs in performance measurement reflects an emphasis on face and content validity. With the exception of some risk-adjustment systems that are used to predict mortality or other reliably measured outcomes, relatively few published research studies on performance measurement in healthcare show evidence of construct or predictive validity. However, to classify these risk-adjustment or severity indexing approaches as *performance measurement systems,* may be to extend their definition beyond that which originally intended by their developers. These approaches are more properly viewed, we believe, as technologies that can assist performance measurement systems to risk- or severity-adjust their measures.

What, then, are the *statistical* characteristics or *indicators* of reliable and valid performance measures? One statistical *indicator* is the shape of the distribution of the rates for the performance measure. Normal or bell-shaped curve approximations are preferred but are in the minority among the host of healthcare performance or outcome measures. Some exceptions in the current arena of process or outcomes measurement, however, are Cesarean delivery rates, total inpatient mortality rates, and overall readmission rates. A few *continuous* measures also are likely to have distributions that approximate the normal curve. These include process measures that look at time until treatment is initiated or the patient is seen, for example, time from emergency department arrival to administration of thrombolytic therapy for confirmed AMI patients, and emergency department wait times. What all these measures have in common is that they are derived from frequently occurring events that are, at present, relatively easy to quantify. Most, if not all of them, involve *content* which not only appears (face validity) to be related to desirable health outcomes but is in fact associated with certain desirable outcomes as shown by credible research (predictive validity).

Events that occur relatively infrequently, if they are reliably reported over a considerable length of time and involve a large sample of participants, may also yield performance measures with desirable psychometric properties. However, one could certainly debate whether or not the term *efficient* should apply to such measures. They may be statistically valid for long-term historical trending of performance but invalid for making inferences about relatively recent phenomena.

Skewed distributions can contain useful data that are reliably measured and validly interpreted. To avoid misuse of statistics, it is important that the appropriate measures of central tendency and variation be used for skewed or Poisson distributions. Medians and percentiles sometimes work better than means and standard deviations for such distributions.

# REFERENCES

1. Adorno, T. W., D. Frenkel-Brunswick, J. Levinson, and R. N. Sanford. 1950. *The authoritarian personality.* New York: Harper.

2. Aron, C. C., D. L. Harper, L. B. Shepardson, and G. E. Rosenthal. 1998. Impact of risk-adjusting Cesarean delivery rates when reporting hospital performance. *JAMA.* 279(24):1968–1972.

3. Bailey, D. 1971. *Probability and statistics.* New York: John Wiley.

4. Brennan, T. A. 1991. Incidence of adverse events and negligence in hospitalized patients: results of the Harvard medical practice study I. *New England Journal of Medicine.* 324(6):370–376.

5. Campbell, D. T., and D. W. Fiske. 1959. Convergent and discriminant validation by the multitrait-multimethod matrix. *Psychological Bulletin.* 56:81–105.

6. Cronbach, L. J. 1951. Coefficient alpha and the internal structure of tests. *Psychometrika.* 16:297–334.

7. Cronbach, L. J., and P. E. Meehl. 1955. Construct validity in psychological tests. *Psychological Bulletin.* 4:281–302.

8. Garcia-Martin, M., et al. 1997. Proportion of hospital deaths associated with adverse events. *J. Clinical Epidemiology.* 50(12):1319–1326.

9. Goldfield, N., and P. Boland. 1996. *Physician profiling and risk adjustment.* Gaithersburg: Aspen Publishers, Inc.

10. Iezzoni, L., ed. 1994. *Risk adjustment for measuring health care outcomes.* Ann Arbor: Health Administration Press.

11. Iezzoni, L. 1997. The risks of risk adjustment. *JAMA.* 270(20):1600–1607.

12. Iezzoni, L., A. Ash, M. Shwartz, et al. 1996. Judging hospitals by severity-adjusted mortality rates. *Am. J. Public Health.* 86:1379–1387.

13. Landon, B., L. Iezzoni, A. Ash, et al. 1996. Judging hospitals by severity-adjusted mortality rates: the case of CABG surgery. *Inquiry.* 33:155–166.

14. Leape, L. L. 1991. The nature of adverse events in hospitalized patients: results of the Harvard medical practice study II. *New England Journal of Medicine.* 324(6):377–384.

15. Winer, B. 1971. *Statistical principles in experimental design.* 2d ed. New York: McGraw-Hill.

# 5

# Data Sources and the Unit of Analysis: The Foundations of Performance Measurement

## THE BASIC *STUFF* OF PERFORMANCE MEASURES

A performance measurement system is rooted in its data sources, which represent the basic *structure* of performance measures. No performance measurement system, no matter how sophisticated its methodologies, can be any better than its foundation data sources. The threatening possibility of form without substance is a factor to be recognized in performance measurement. This fact is sometimes obscured in this information age of fabulous technology where 3-D graphics and hypertext often create the illusion of substance.

The foundations of performance measurement systems, their fundamental structures and architecture, are riveted to three generic categories of data.

- Medical records data—derived from data elements abstracted from medical records or some other related data source

- Administrative data—derived from large, computerized files used in billing health services

- Patient data—data derived from information collected directly from patients through interviews, surveys, or inventories. Some examples are patient satisfaction surveys and health status profile questionnaires

## Medical Records Data

The collection of medical records data is often based on reservations about the clinical content of administrative data (Iezzoni, 1994). Many performance measurement systems rely in part or almost exclusively on clinical data elements available from the patient's medical record and/or related data sources such as infection control records and laboratory results. Medical records vary widely in their quality. Medical records and the clinical content derived from them are potentially rich in information about the patient. At their very best, they provide a comprehensive picture of the patient. At their worst, medical records are incomplete, inaccurate, and dominated by subjectivity. The data derived from them will suffer accordingly. New computer technologies, the ability to enter clinical data directly online, and the appreciation of the need for clinically rich data are all contributing to increased use of medical records data in measuring performance. Medical records data, in combination with the two data sources which follow—administrative and patient—offer the best prospect for a comprehensive and content-valid approach to performance measurement in healthcare.

## Administrative Data

Administrative data are derived from claims or other mandated records. Since these databases are primarily designed to pay claims (reimburse providers), they are not readily amenable for use in performance measurement. One of the other drawbacks is lack of timeliness, particularly for administrative data based on claims. Currently, it can take three months or longer to pay a claim, and complete data for a particular time period may not be available until many months after the services are rendered. Those attempting to measure provider performance must decide whether to accept incomplete data and report the results in timely fashion or to wait until all of the data are available and report results months after the fact. Neither approach is completely tenable in the current healthcare environment. It is misleading to report on the basis of incomplete data and not very meaningful to report provider data months after the fact. Still, there are advantages and disadvantages to administrative data in developing performance measures. Administrative data collected as a requirement of reimbursement are uniformly generated and can offer a population-based data source when denominator information is available (Retchin & Ballard, 1998). These measures use data that are relatively available and affordable, even if they are not usually timely. They do not require additional resources involved in gathering data (medical records and laboratory results) which are abstracted. The data are available at the patient level and can be cleaned and edited using internally or externally developed methods designed specifically for these data. The databases are usually well designed—at least for their primary purpose—and have a *history of usage*. Such a history tends to be associated with increased reliability and accuracy of reporting. With unique identifiers, such databases provide the possibility of following patients throughout their continuum of care.

A final strength of administrative data sets is their amenability to computerized risk-adjustment technologies; several risk- or severity-adjustment software systems have been designed for administrative data sets with a measure of success. However, *success* is often dampened by the fact that administrative data may reflect patient conditions that were a consequence of treatments received during a current episode of care, not conditions that were present upon admission. This factor may invalidate the risk-adjustment methodology. In addition, administrative data often lack clinical face validity—useful or not, they may not be credible to clinicians. Since they are focused primarily on cost and utilization, they may lack content validity—the *richness of content* that is available from some forms of nonadministrative data.

There are many current efforts to expand and improve administrative data sets. A number of emerging privately owned performance measurement systems are based solely on administrative data elements. Other private vendors have purchased and used administrative data sets in sophisticated arrangements, linking records to other data sets (patient functional status, hospital cost data). The terminology, data definitions, coding, and general content of administrative data are well known by most professionals in health services research. As a consequence of the ubiquity of administrative data sets, results based on the analysis of these data are easily understood and communicated among clinical practitioners, researchers, administrators, and organizations—virtually guaranteeing their continued use.

## Patient Data

Patient data include questionnaire or survey information obtained directly from patients or from caretakers or others who are familiar with the patients. Among the primary areas comprising patient data in health services are patient satisfaction, health status, functional status, and patient preferences. These measures are fundamentally different from administrative and medical record data in that they are much more amenable to well-developed psychometric methods of assessing their reliability and validity. Most of these measures are in the form of items, which are scored. Frequently the data are *ordinal* which means that some value can be assigned to them on an ordered scale. At the lowest level in terms of ordinal measurement are items or checklists subject to 0 or 1 scoring (*no* or *yes* responses). At a higher level, in terms of measurement attributes, are items scored along a continuum; the level of measurement is termed *interval,* since, theoretically, there are equal measured intervals between the value points for such items. For example, responses to an item varying on a five-point scale from *strongly disagree* to *strongly agree* usually comprise *equal-interval* measurement. The responses cannot only be ordered in terms of value but the orderings are of equal distance from one another along the underlying dimension or construct that is being measured.

It is possible to assess reliability and validity for such measures through multiple methods. Patients can be tested and then retested and their test results correlated in order to determine stability of scores over time, one way of actually measuring reliability. Alternatively, one can measure the correlation coefficients among the items of a survey or questionnaire if results are available on a sufficient number of patients in order to determine the measure's *internal consistency,* another form of reliability assessment. Does the measure correlate with other similar measures? Is the measure essentially unrelated to other measures that are based on fundamentally different constructs? These are the types of questions related to validity that are frequently addressed and often satisfactorily answered when the scientific methods employed by statisticians and psychometricians are used in analyzing patient data.

At their best, patient data are probably the most reliable and valid of all three data types—at least from the point of view of psychometric assessment. This may seem surprising to some since such data often seem to be too subjective and biased to be valid. While these data may be subject to all sorts of influences such as *social desirability* (Crown & Marlowe, 1964), malingering, faking, *demand characteristics,* or other *response sets,* they have the advantage of being *multiply measured.* As seen by psychometricians, administrative data and medical records data are essentially one-item measures of some underlying construct purportedly measured, whether it be cost, quality, or some other variable. While one item may be sufficient to measure cost—cost just needs to be reported accurately—one item may not be sufficient to measure something as abstract as *quality*. For such abstractions, if the item attempting to measure the abstraction fails, the entire measure fails. The item-test may not fail per se, but it may not take into account the totality of what it purports to measure. In short, the item-test lacks content validity.

Patient-derived data, on the other hand, usually contain a number of items for each dimension measured. The advantages of multiple item scales over single item scales are threefold: higher reliability, greater scope, and more precision (Nunnally & Bernstein, 1994). The untoward effects of poor items are often negated by items with good reliability and validity. In addition, through item analysis, one can improve the measure by eliminating poor items.

Psychometrics, which has benefited greatly from the exigencies of educational placement and personnel selection over most of this century, has greatly contributed to the usefulness of patient data in the health sciences. Somewhat paradoxically, patient-derived data, while the most *subjective* in content, are, perhaps, the most *objective* of the three data types in terms of their measurement status. The methods of continuous quality improvement (CQI) are readily adapted to patient measures. In fact, while infrequently discussed in the context of CQI, many of the methods applied to patient data are consistent with CQI concepts. The advent of the *information age,* the development of high-speed microprocessors, and the availability of user-friendly statistical software have dramatically shortened the time of conducting the necessary iterative processes in the development and revision of patient-derived measures. Such iterative processes mirror the methods of CQI.

One of the most common criticisms of patient data in the health services arena, particularly where quality is concerned, is that patients are often perceived as poor judges of the quality of medical care that they receive. There is reason to believe that many patients lack realistic expectations regarding the probable outcome of medical interventions. Limited knowledge of medical options and the appropriateness of various treatments, combined with the probabilistic nature of medicine (Kazandjian, 1995), leave patients confused, frequently fearful, and often less than objective in evaluating the quality of their care. Yet, most patients surveyed in the United States in the 1990s indicate that they are relatively satisfied with their healthcare and their provider. Do these results accurately reflect public sentiments regarding the quality of medical care practiced in this country? This is an interesting question which cannot be answered satisfactorily at present. The manner in which questionnaires and surveys are constructed, how the items are worded, the propensity of patients to respond in a *socially desirable manner,* and other factors influence the results of patient surveys.

We believe that patient data should play an expanded role in measuring performance of healthcare providers, particularly if there is increased interest in the health status of patients in the community. Even if patients are poor judges of quality of care, which is debatable, the growing competition among providers and health plans will assure that health status, patient satisfaction, and other patient factors are assessed. Patient data remain valuable, especially when combined with other types of data (administrative, medical records) in measuring provider performance.

## THE UNIT OF ANALYSIS: INDIVIDUALS, GROUPS, OR ORGANIZATIONS

As we discussed, the data source of a performance measure can affect the types of conclusions (and the confidence we have in them) that can be derived from the measure. Similarly, the implications that can be derived from a performance measure are quite different, depending on the measure's unit of analysis. The *unit of analysis,* whether it be individuals, groups, or organizations, is, therefore, as important as the data sources of the performance measure in determining the performance measure's ultimate utility. As discussed in an earlier chapter, we believe that the science of individual measurement is relatively well developed. On the other hand, *with the exception of the financial performance and easily quantified measures of organizational output,* in our opinion, the sciences of group and organizational measurement—especially in the healthcare arena—while emerging are still relatively embryonic.

Since our main interest is with the measurement of performance in organizations—more specifically, healthcare organizations—the developmental nature of this field as a scientific discipline poses some problems, but it also provides opportunities. The field of performance measurement in healthcare, in general, still lacks standard definitions, and there is little agreement as to what performance is outside of the financial arena. There are hundreds of *performance measurement systems* which, more or less, tap similar domains of performance content, but there have been a dearth of systematic studies that have appeared in peer review publications addressing how well these systems measure whatever it is they measure. Most of the current performance measures, no matter what system they comprise, have varying degrees of *face validity* (the extent to which a measure appears to be valid). Evidence for other forms of validity (content, construct, predictive) are usually not to be found. Evidence of reliability (consistency of measurement), a precursor for validity, is also often lacking.

To some extent, the lack of evidence of reliability and validity in many performance measures used by healthcare organizations can be attributed to the relatively undeveloped state of performance measurement in healthcare. Few systems have been around more than a decade or so, and it takes time and resources to establish reliability and validity. The emphasis has clearly been on developing measures that are not too difficult to implement or too draining on the resources of healthcare organizations. Reliable and valid measures take time to develop, involve extensive and intensive training of users, and must be implemented carefully and consistently if the results are to be used to compare performance among a number of organizations. Moreover, reliable and valid measures must not only be well designed, they must be based on definitions that are uniformly applied. Again, this necessitates a commitment on the part of the user (the healthcare organization) to assure quality reporting; it also requires that the performance measurement system monitor or audit the users to make sure that reporting is consistent with established standards.

A case can be made that the measurement of group and organizational performance, for the most part, has been based on a fundamentally different paradigm than that of the measurement of individuals, especially the measurement of *individual differences.* If so, are these paradigms different by necessity or by accident? Do they simply reflect differences in the state of nature (or the phenomena being measured) or do they reflect differences in approaches which are mainly arbitrary? Is it possible to take a *middle ground* on this issue of different paradigms— a position that suggests that group and organizational measurement can be enhanced by adopting some of the approaches commonly used in individual measurement and vice versa? While we cannot answer these questions, we can at least provide a context and present some elements to consider in addressing the underlying issues.

# INDIVIDUAL MEASUREMENT AND ASSESSMENT OF ORGANIZATIONAL PERFORMANCE

### Health Status

There is at least one area which is ripe (in organizational performance) for applying the techniques of individual (patient) assessment, namely, health status. There are several measures of health status reported in the literature. One of the most widely used measures of health status is the SF-36™ Health Survey (Ware et al., 1993).[1] This 36-item survey was developed in order to meet minimum psychometric standards necessary for group comparisons involving generic health concepts. Many of the items on this questionnaire are based on instruments in use for more than 20 years. A 149-item "Functioning and Well-Being Profile" (Stewart & Ware, 1992) served as the source for the 36 items in the survey. The SF-36™ has been well tested for both reliability (internal consistency and test-retest) and validity (content, concurrent, criterion, construct, and predictive). The SF-36™ measures health status in the following eight areas: physical functioning, role functioning (physical), bodily pain, general health, vitality, social functioning, role functioning (emotional), and mental health. The SF-36™ has been used to assess health status in a variety of patient conditions including but not limited to the following: hip replacement (Katz et al., 1992), asthma (Bousquet et al., 1994), epilepsy (Hermann, 1995), cardiac disease (Jette & Downing, 1994), stroke (Kappelle et al., 1994), and diabetes (Jacobsen et al., 1994).

### OASIS

Another prominent measure of individual health-related behaviors used to assess organizational performance (home health agencies) is the Outcome and Assessment Information Set (OASIS-B) developed by the University of Colorado's Center for Health Policy Research (1997). The OASIS is a 79-item survey (completed by the home health agency caregiver) which measures several dimensions of individual health status and functioning including living arrangements; supportive assistance; sensory, integumentary, respiratory, elimination, and neuro/emotional/behavioral status; activities of daily living (ADLs); medications; equipment management; and emergent care. The Health Care Finance Administration (HCFA) has pro-

---

[1] A briefer version of this survey is also available: the SF-12™.

posed that the OASIS be completed on Medicare patients served by home health agencies as a condition for participating in the Medicare program.

## Patient Satisfaction

In addition to health status and functioning surveys, patient satisfaction questionnaires have been used to assess organizational performance. One of the most prominent patient satisfaction surveys is the 52-item Picker/Commonwealth Survey (Picker, 1992). The Picker/Commonwealth Survey elicits information about the following dimensions of patient satisfaction: physical support, emotional support, communication, needs and preferences, pain management, financial factors, family participation, education, and discharge preparation. Another widely used instrument to assess patient satisfaction is the Group Health Association of America (GHAA) Survey (Davies & Ware, 1991). This survey has 60 items covering various dimensions of patient satisfaction including general satisfaction with care, satisfaction with services and providers, satisfaction with health insurance and the use of services, satisfaction with the health plan, and satisfaction with personal characteristics. The GHAA Survey has demonstrated internal consistency, reliability, and validity (face, predictive) when used to assess managed care plans.

## Assessing Organizations Through Individual Assessment

*The measurement of group and organizational performance based on methods developed for individual assessment (health status, functional status, patient satisfaction) appears to be gaining momentum.* Many psychometrically sound instruments are available, and, often, these instruments can be adapted or modified for the specific organizations or groups being researched. Of course, the remaining question is a potentially contentious one: Should we hold healthcare organizations responsible for the health status, health functioning, and satisfaction of the individuals they serve? We believe that this question has been already answered by the number of initiatives in these areas. Whether healthcare organizations can be held accountable for the health status of the communities they serve is another issue. Consider the fact, however, that many healthcare organizations are being transformed into comprehensive integrated delivery systems by consolidating and/or merging on a grand scale. An argument can be made that such integrated delivery systems, by serving entire communities, should be held accountable (at least in part) for the health status of the members of those communities. This sort of accountability has been given impetus by the Healthy People 2000 initiative in the form of various health status objectives for the United States.[2]

## Future of Individual Assessment Techniques Vis-à-Vis the Organization

One of the greatest impediments to the wide adoption of individual measurement methodologies to assess group and organizational performance is cost. Other issues to consider before embarking in such efforts include confidentiality, patient literacy, logistics, and tracking. Despite some drawbacks, we believe that the methodologies of individual assessment will find increasingly more application in group and organizational performance assessment. These approaches have the inherent advantage of measuring what is most directly affecting patients—their health status, their level of functioning, and their perceptions about the care they receive. In addition, many of these methodologies have demonstrated reliability and validity in accord with generally accepted psychometric standards. The ability to collect, process, analyze, and report data of this type has been greatly enhanced by development of new data management technologies. While in the past such processing capabilities were only available with large mainframe computers, the desk top computer now has enough *power* to perform the necessary operations involved in this type of large-scale processing. An abundance of user-friendly statistical software is available for a *windows* environment, allowing researchers to do their own programming without relying on other professionals trained in more traditional programming applications. For all these reasons, we believe that individual measurement of health status, functioning, and perceptions about care will increasingly dominate the performance measurement arena in the next decade.

## Observation and Experimentation

This topic may seem more relevant in an introductory textbook in the physical or social sciences than it does in a book about performance measurement. It is, however, our observation that there is not enough consideration about the assumptions we make about these processes when we measure performance—how they are alike, how they differ, and the types

---

[2] Facilitated by the U.S. Federal Government, this work has been termed "a statement of national opportunities."

of inferences we can legitimately draw from them. We begin by defining these terms.

*Observation.* the process of *watching* or perceiving the detail and/or *gestalt* of events so that the events can be described or recorded. Under this definition, *watching* can be done with not only our eyes but with any sense organ; for example, we can *watch* with our ears when faced with auditory phenomena or with our nose when faced with olfactory phenomena.

*Experimentation.* a controlled observation (or set of controlled observations) in which we set out to test one or more hypotheses or theories by varying one or more conditions, holding others constant (not allowing them to vary), and evaluate the results using unbiased methods. The key to this definition is the term *controlled* which refers to the fact that we vary one or more sets of factors (experimental treatments) and hold all other factors constant—we allow only those factors we are investigating to vary.

Observation is a necessary but not sufficient condition for experimentation. Observation, alone, implies no attempt to intervene in events; we simply *observe* what is happening, and, if we are good observers, we may be able to draw some tentative inferences from our observations. There is nothing intrinsically scientific about observation, but it is clear that all science begins with observation. Once again, we can *observe* with our ears or any sense organ, just as we *observe* with our eyes.

It is hard to conceive of a science with no experimental component. Science is rooted in both exploration and confirmation. Observation is the basis of hypothesis or theory generation, while experimentation is the basis of hypothesis or theory testing. Observation is *exploratory,* while experimentation is *confirmatory.*

### Do We Meet the Rigors of a Scientific Discipline?

In most current applications, when we measure performance in healthcare, are we engaging in anything beyond a detailed observation of healthcare events? If not, can we say that our measurement is *scientific?* These are critical questions that deserve attention. There are, of course, numerous examples of the application of experimental science in healthcare. One such example is randomized, controlled studies in which the effects of treatments (factors, conditions) are compared using random assignment of subjects to treatment groups. In most applications of performance measurement, however, the stringent demands of randomized, controlled studies are not met. Patients are not often randomly assigned to healthcare organizations in order to compare outcomes among healthcare organizations.

Various techniques to control extraneous sources of variation, some based on risk and severity-adjustment methods, have been developed and widely implemented to compare performance among organizations. Fundamentally, these approaches are designed to neutralize the effects of factors that are differentially distributed among providers of healthcare but related to healthcare outcomes or *performance.* Social scientists use similar techniques in attempting to control factors that are related to the dependent variable but unequally distributed between the experimental and control groups. In the healthcare arena, there is recent evidence that such approaches have not been as useful as had been anticipated (Iezzoni, 1997).

Essentially, then, performance measurement which is designed to compare organizations does not meet the rigorous requirements of an *experimental science,* if that term denotes randomized controlled studies. This is not to say that the measures are not scientific; rather it is the methodology in its totality that falls short of what we call *hard science.* Various adjustments, which serve as substitutes for the experimental controls of hard science, have not demonstrated sufficient validity over a range of conditions to elevate the methodologies of performance measurement to the level dictated by experimental science.

### Why Does Organizational Performance Measurement Fall Short as an Experimental Science?

Organizational performance measurement, generally speaking, usually occurs as detailed observation relying on instruments with various levels of precision. Lack of instrument precision can be ameliorated somewhat (by increasing the sample size and/or by risk-adjusting), but it cannot be completely eliminated since the methodology is essentially observational. *Why is it that an experimental science of organizational performance measurement has not developed?* This question involves at least four considerations: ethics, costs, logistics, and politics.

### Ethical Concerns

Restricting patients' choices or outright denial of some forms of healthcare raises ethical concerns, whether these limitations are undertaken in an experimental situation or *laboratory* with patients' signed approval or in a field setting, with or without patient approval. Random assignment of patients (subjects) to different providers of care (or healthcare organizations) becomes an ethical issue if patients are not fully informed about the terms and conditions of the study. Patients with any kind of condition, no matter how serious or how minor, have a right to seek care from the best providers of care. In randomized, controlled studies, there is often an array of treatments (with suspected or well-documented varying degrees of efficacy) along with a control group in which there is no treatment or a *placebo treatment*. Patients agreeing to participate in these studies are made aware of these factors—that they may receive a placebo or a minimally effective treatment. Safeguards of this type are difficult to implement in naturalistic or field settings in which different providers of care become the *treatments*. Without such safeguards, getting approval to do experimental research in which there is *random assignment of patients to providers of care* is rare.

### Costs Issues

Even if ethical concerns can somehow be satisfied, the costs of performing *highly controlled* field research in which patients are randomly assigned to different providers of care (or organizations) can be prohibitive. Almost all highly controlled field research studies are expensive for a number of reasons: they are frequently very large-scale, involve a lot of participants, and involve extensive follow-up in community settings. It is this last reason that presents the greatest unknown in terms of costs. Following up patients for one or two weeks post-discharge is one thing, for a year or more, quite another. Many studies require follow-up for as long as five years or more such as long-term outcomes following cardiac surgery.

### Logistics

Experimental studies involving large healthcare organizations frequently require extensive follow-up of patients. It is often difficult to do an adequate follow-up of patients after they are discharged—at least, to do follow-up that is comprehensive, extends over a meaningful period of time, and yields credible data. Patient attrition comes in three forms: the patient dies, moves and cannot be reached, or drops out of the study for some other reason. Unless mortality is one of the dependent variables—which, of course, is common in healthcare research—patient mortality has negative consequences for the study. The other forms of attrition can also detract from the research effort. Conclusions are more tentative due to incomplete data or worse. For example, did the patient drop out because of one of the interventions or was the attrition completely independent of the intervention? Since the patient is ipso facto unavailable, the question usually cannot be answered.

Issues of continuity relating to research philosophy, procedures, and personnel also impact the study's ability to collect consistent data over an extensive time period. Turnover in the research team, changes in data collection procedures, and *mid-stream* changes in the underlying assumptions of the study (often philosophically based due to changes in leadership) can singularly or in combination have a huge impact on the results of the study. Some of these changes may be unavoidable and some may even improve the study. However, they have to be taken into account when extensive follow-up of patients is required.

### The Ubiquity of Politics

Political considerations can dominate the debate when an attempt is made to compare outcomes among different organizations. Who can see the data? What can they see? When can they see it? These questions apply even if the research is not experimental in the sense that we are using it here.

There is growing pressure on healthcare organizations to report performance data. This pressure primarily stems from the influences of employer groups, consumer advocates, regulatory agencies, and managed care organizations. Some healthcare organizations, including *health plans,* have responded to these pressures by releasing performance data to the public. How useful these data have been to consumers in terms of decision making regarding healthcare is still an open issue. Without a proper *context,* such data can be misleading. In some managed care plans, healthcare consumers (enrollees) are given an opportunity to select their managed care organizations (MCOs). This kind of arrangement makes it possible to compare outcomes by MCO. The results can be useful—especially if there is an attempt to control for group differences by risk or severity-adjustment; but this methodology does not meet the criteria of an experimental science. Consumer rights and the perceived benefits of patient choice still far outweigh, as they should, other considerations in the public politic.

# REFERENCES

1. Bousquet, J., J. Knani, H. Dhivert, et al. 1994. Quality of life in asthma: I. internal consistency and validity of the SF-36 Questionnaire. *American Journal of Respiratory and Critical Care Medicine.* 149:371–375.

2. Crown, D. P., and D. Marlowe. 1964. *The approval motive.* New York: John Wiley.

3. Davies, A., and J. Ware. 1991. *GHAA's Consumer Satisfaction Survey and User's Manual.* Washington, D.C.: Group Health Association of America.

4. *Healthy People 2000: National Health Promotion and Disease Prevention Objectives.* 1991. U.S. Department of Health and Human Services: Public Health Service. Washington: U.S. Government Printing Office.

5. Hermann, B. 1995. The evolution of health-related quality of life assessment in epilepsy. *Qual. Life Res.* 4:87–100.

6. Iezzoni, L. I., ed. 1994. *Risk adjustment for measuring health care outcomes.* Ann Arbor: Health Administration Press.

7. Jacobsen A., M. De Grott, and J. Samson. 1994. The evaluation of two measures of quality of life in patients with type I and type II diabetes. *Diabetes Care.* 17(4):267–274.

8. Jette, D., and J. Downing. 1994. Health status of individuals entering a cardiac rehabilitation program as measured by the Medical Outcomes Study 36-Item Short-Form Survey (SF-36). *Physical Therapy.* 74(6):521–527.

9. Kappelle L., H. Adams, M. Heffner, J. Torner, F. Gomez, and J. Biller. 1994. Prognosis of young adults with ischemic stroke: a long-term follow-up study assessing recurrent vascular events and functional outcome in the Iowa Registry of Stroke in young adults. *Stroke.* 25(7):1360–1365.

10. Katz, J., T. Harris, and M. Larson. 1992. Predictors of functional outcomes after arthroscopic partial meniscetomy. *Journal of Rheumatology.* 19(12):1938–1942.

11. Kazandjian, V. K. 1995. The future of outcomes research may benefit from the evolution of medical critical thinking. *The Joint Commission Journal of Quality Improvement.* 21(10):553–557.

12. *Medicare Home Health Care Quality Assurance and Improvement Demonstration Outcome and Assessment Information Set (OASIS-B).* 1997. Denver: Center for Health Policy Research.

13. Nunnally, J. C., and I. H. Bernstein. 1994. *Psychometric Theory.* 3d ed. New York: McGraw-Hill.

14. *Picker/Commonwealth Hospital Satisfaction Survey.* 1992. Picker Institute.

15. Retchin, S. M., and D. J. Ballard. 1998. Commentary: establishing standards for the utility of administrative claims data. *Health Services Research.* 32(6):861–866.

16. Stewart, A., and J. Ware. 1992. *Measuring functioning and well-being: the medical outcomes study approach.* Durham: Duke University Press.

17. Ware, J. E., K. K. Snow, M. Kosinski, and B. Gandek. 1993. *SF-36 Health Survey Manual and Interpretation Guide.* Boston: New England Medical Center, The Health Institute.

# The Hawthorne Studies Revisited: Implications for Performance Measurement in the Information Age

The significance of the Hawthorne studies can be understood not only in relation to their findings but also because they are an outstanding example of research that was not steered to predetermined conclusions and because they raised questions that otherwise might not have been asked. (Milton Blum & James Naylor, 1968)

## BACKGROUND

Research in the laboratory and the field contains numerous examples of the *serendipity factor.* The serendipity factor occurs when good things are found accidentally. The researcher sets out to test one set of hypotheses and discovers new things unrelated or only obliquely related to the initial assumptions of the study. This situation of serendipity occurred in the legendary and now classic Hawthorne studies (Rothlesberger & Dixon, 1939). These studies continue to be reexamined in terms of the intellectual and political dynamics of the experiments and their evolution from tentative experimentation to seemingly authoritative publications (Gillespie, 1993).

It was the openness of the researchers—their lack of preconceived notions—that allowed the Hawthorne researchers to see beyond their initial assumptions and to take advantage of the *serendipity factor.* The Hawthorne studies may seem *dated* to some readers. They obviously occurred during a time that our culture was still very much immersed in the industrial age. The information age would not appear on the horizon for two decades after the conclusion of the Hawthorne studies. Even so, a brief review of the initial assumptions of this research, its methods, and, at that time, its surprising results, can tell us something about performance measurement.

## THE HAWTHORNE STUDIES REVISITED

The Hawthorne studies were, in reality, five interrelated studies conducted by Harvard University and the Western Electric Company between 1927 and 1937 at its Hawthorne plant in Illinois. The research was initially guided by three assumptions regarding the relationship between industrial organization and efficiency.

- Factory organization is fundamentally a technological problem.

- Man is rationale and, therefore, primarily motivated by economic incentives.

- Given appropriate economic incentives, production is a simple function of objective working conditions and individual constitutional factors.

---

### The Hawthorne Studies Summarized: First Study

In the first study, experiments on illumination, the production of workers varied without any direct relationship to the amount of illumination—contrary to the experimenters' assumptions. The anomalous results of this study would have discouraged many investigators, causing an early end to the experiment. The Hawthorne investigators, however, believed that there was something to be learned from these strange findings.

---

### Second Study

In the second study, relay assembly test room, the experimenters concluded that there was a relationship between employee morale and supervision practices (all employees were women in this study). However, they found that they could not predict the effects of any given variable if it were part of a total situation. After the second study, the experimenters realized that more knowledge was needed about the workers and their attitudes.

## Third Study

The third study was set up to determine how to improve supervision. The approach that was used was a massive employee interview program using the indirect method of interview. Repeatedly, employees claimed to have benefited from the opportunity to freely express themselves. One of the most significant findings of the third study was the effect that informal groups had on individual worker attitudes and behavior—groups not recognized formally by the organization. It was clear that such groups can and do set limits on production; they also influence worker attitudes, for better or worse, which can affect turnover, absenteeism, and other job-related factors.

## Fourth Study

The bank wiring observation room, the fourth study, was undertaken to obtain more information about the informal or social groups within the company. In this study, it was uncovered that bank wiring observation room employees (all men) devised various means of controlling production (restricting output) including name calling and minor physical punishment. The men were able to keep weekly production fairly constant by reporting more work than actually produced on some days and less work than actually produced on other days. Communications traveled down in the form of orders, but there was a gap in communications from bottom to the top, which in this case, was the foreman level. The organization of cliques was based on four sets of beliefs about work: (1) there should not be too much production or *rate-busting*, (2) there should not be too little production or *chiseling*, (3) there should be no *squealing*—telling supervisors anything that would harm an associate, and (4) there should be no *officious* work behaviors, either on the part of workers or supervisors. This intricate social organization protected the group from both inside and outside forces (Blum & Naylor, 1968).

## Fifth Study

The fifth and final study was *personnel counseling,* the most practical of the five studies. The fifth study had two objectives: (1) to conduct an impartial interview of employees to gain an understanding of their problems and help supervisors improve their methods of supervision and (2) to improve communications within the company, especially in those areas in which the goals of the informal social organization were in conflict with those of management. To meet these objectives, personnel men were assigned to departments and were available to the employees for discussion of work matters. Overall, the personnel counseling program was accepted by the employees and was credited as improving three areas of concern to management and employees: employee-management relations, supervisor-employee relations, and personal adjustment.

It needs to be stated that the Hawthorne studies were less than ideal in terms of experimental design; there were a number of methodological biases in these studies. For example, some of the differences in findings between the second and fourth studies might be explained by the fact that the second study contained all women and the fourth study, all men. Despite these and other shortcomings, the Hawthorne studies made an important contribution to social, management, economic, and health sciences. They are unique, especially for the period in which they occurred, in that they were utterly focused on what it is that people do—observing and recording behaviors without yielding to any vested academic interests or ideologies. Perhaps the achievements of the Hawthorne studies are best summarized by Hart (1942). In referring to the experimenters, he states:

> They stuck to what happens and therefore could never allow themselves or their work to be compartmentalized. And just because they refused to compartmentalize, all the compartments have something to learn from them.
>
> There is no label that can be put on these experiments because they are experiments in a unique field, the field of real human beings. Before Rothlesberger and his colleagues, few had dared to enter that untrodden territory; in modern cultures none had dared.

## IMPLICATIONS FOR PERFORMANCE MEASUREMENT SYSTEMS

The *Hawthorne effect* is now used to describe the positive impact on behavior that sometimes occurs in a study or experiment as a result of the interest shown by the experimenter in the humans who are being treated, studied, or observed. The positive impact on performance is temporary, ending as soon as attitudes return to their normal state. The observed improvement is, thus, the result of attitudinal change, not the experimental *treatment* per se.

One of the most important implications for healthcare from the Hawthorne studies is that in any health intervention we are first and foremost dealing with human beings, both as providers and as recipients of care. While this may seem obvious, the ramifications of this simple statement of fact can be forgotten when we start talking about structures, processes, outcomes, risk-adjustments, clinical pathways, and the like. Such terms, while useful and necessary, can sometimes obscure the very fundamental fact that healthcare is about human beings doing something to (or making decisions about) other human beings.

When we conduct research in healthcare, the level of human involvement is especially complex. In this arena, we have researchers interacting with providers of care who, in turn, interact with patients. Who are the experimental subjects in this situation? Are they the providers of care, or are they the recipients of care? We propose that the *experimental subjects* under this scenario are both the recipients and providers of care.

> *Whether we acknowledge it or not, when we measure performance we are performing a kind of intervention.*

The very act of measuring alters that which is measured (Heisenberg Principle). The results of the measurements are used to make decisions about structures and processes of care—or, if you like, about how well human beings are caring for other human beings. Human actions (processes) lead to outcomes which can be measured and interpreted, ultimately leading to decisions about modification of processes or maintaining the status quo.

The *Hawthorne effect* can assert itself in at least two ways in this set of circumstances. The providers of care are impacted by the treatment directly—which, in this case, is the act of measurement—and the recipients of care are impacted directly or indirectly by the measurement-intervention. The *Hawthorne effect* is manifested by temporary improvements in attitudes by either providers of care, patients, or both leading to transient changes in processes of care and patient outcomes.

When we review the Hawthorne studies and their implications for performance measurement, two questions immediately come to mind: How can we separate the *Hawthorne effect* from *real change?* As long as there is improvement, do we care if it is solely the result of the Hawthorne effect?

# THE HAWTHORNE EFFECT vs. *REAL CHANGE*

The Hawthorne effect is usually temporary. Can we distinguish between results attributable to Hawthorne factors and those attributable to the intended intervention (*real change*) or to the *placebo effect*,[1] for that

---

[1] According to the Shorter Oxford Dictionary, the term *placebo* has been used since 1811 to mean a medicine given more to please than to benefit a patient. The *placebo effect* refers to the fact that medicine and other treatments lacking *active ingredients* can have a beneficial effect on patients. This effect has been well documented in medical research.

matter. Some problems have solutions that transcend language, and our *literacy* may get in the way of helping us differentiate Hawthorne effects from those effects resulting from intended interventions or from placebos. Perhaps a change in paradigm is necessary. The situation can be especially complex when the *treatment* is an initiative such as *continuous quality improvement* (CQI), an approach that tends to foster attitude change yielding improved performance along the same lines as the Hawthorne effect.

*One possible way of identifying a Hawthorne effect is by its temporality—* Hawthorne effects wear off quickly. Many interventions, including CQI, may have long-lasting or *quasi-permanent* effects, depending on circumstances. A second means of distinguishing Hawthorne from other effects may be to ask the *subjects,* whoever they are, to explain the causes of their improved performance. Their responses can sometimes identify whether or not it was the intervention per se that resulted in the improved performance or factors related to *sentiments,* a term that was frequently used by the Hawthorne investigators to explain anomalous results.

## CAPITALIZING ON INITIAL POSITIVE ATTITUDES

*The initial change in attitudes commonly found in research studies (the Hawthorne effect) can be used by designers of performance measurement systems to help them reach their overall goals.* The Hawthorne effect does not have to be viewed strictly as a confounding factor in performance measurement. In some cases, the Hawthorne effect can be used to the advantage of designers of performance measurement systems in trying to get a new measurement system successfully promoted. A new, but well-designed performance measurement system may well need a *jump start* to gain respectability—or at the very least, a suspension of judgment—a *jump start* that can be achieved by some of the same factors operating in the Hawthorne studies over 60 years ago. *Listening* to people who are (or soon will be) using the new performance measurement system is critical in gaining initial support for that system.

## IMPLICATIONS FOR CHOOSING A PERFORMANCE MEASUREMENT SYSTEM

Whatever the approach to performance measurement, the results ultimately must be validated—by both the methods of direct observation (face validation) and through scientific research. The Hawthorne studies suggest that the best approach to performance measurement and its validation is interdisciplinary—an approach which looks at what it is that healthcare professionals do from various vantage points. This implies that a host of professionals—clinical practitioners, epidemiologists, statisticians, social scientists, economists, and the like—can provide unique perspectives to performance measurement that, in sum, will ultimately lead to better performance indicators. The Hawthorne studies suggest the need to discard concepts that do not fit the empirical data and to revise faulty assumptions *early in the game*. These classic studies would likely have been disbanded after the illumination experiments if the researchers had refused to abandon their initial assumptions. As in the Hawthorne experiments, in developing performance measures for healthcare, it may sometimes be necessary to abandon initial concepts and assumptions—or, if you like, preconceived notions—in order to develop measures that are practical to implement and useful to providers.

## DOES PERFORMANCE MEASUREMENT AFFECT PERFORMANCE?

*There can be no greater justification for performance measurement than its power to impact that which it is measuring.* Yet, the empirical evidence for such impact is scarce in the healthcare arena. There is barely a handful of published studies that have demonstrated or, at least, suggested that performance measurement contributed to improved patient outcomes. These include the inpatient mortality studies of coronary artery bypass graft (CABG) patients in New York, Pennsylvania, and New England as well as the Cesarean section cohort study (Kazandjian & Lied, 1997) of the Maryland Hospital Association's Quality Indicator Project®. One thing all these studies have in common is that they used indicators that are well researched and have found at least a degree of acceptance in the field as reliable and valid measures of performance.

Our fundamental argument is that performance measurement should be subjected to the same scientific scrutiny as any intervention in healthcare. The demonstration of positive impact on processes of care or patient outcomes sets a new standard for performance measurement systems. Currently, the emphasis is on developing systems that report user-friendly performance data on a near real-time basis. Such data are undeniably valuable to healthcare professionals, payers, and regulators, but what some consider their most important purpose in the long run, improving performance, has taken a backseat to data reporting demands. Perhaps users have not fully realized the potential of performance measurement to transcend its customary uses such as tracking performance within organizations or comparing performance against similar organizations for marketing purposes. That said, we believe that healthcare organizations are increasingly using performance data for benchmarking purposes, an application which can lead to improved processes of care and, ultimately, to improved patient outcomes. The urgent demand for benchmarking could, therefore, lead healthcare organizations to *shop around* for performance measures and systems that can scientifically demonstrate a positive impact on processes and outcomes. If such measures are found and successfully adopted, healthcare organizations can meet both their internal quality improvement objectives and external marketing goals.

What kinds of performance measurement systems are most likely to demonstrate a positive impact on processes or outcomes? This question is difficult to answer, at least in the manner in which it is stated. Perhaps a better question is: What are the characteristics of measures that are likely to yield data that can be used to improve processes or outcomes of care? This question suggests yet another question: What are the characteristics of healthcare organizations that are most likely to improve their processes of care and patient outcomes as a result of performance measurement data? To address these related questions, we refer to what can be termed *the symbiosis of measurement and management* and its two axioms: (1) you can't manage what you can't measure (Goonan, 1995) and its less known converse, (2) you can't measure what you can't manage.

### The Symbiosis of Measurement and Management

*You can't manage what you can't measure.* This axiom seems so elementary it's astonishing how often it is violated. Examples of its violation are ubiquitous—ranging from the mundane level of personal financial management to the mega-level of managing multinational resources. In healthcare, we believe that the inability (or unwillingness) to measure what providers of healthcare do, what happens to patients, and the links between providers and patients are root sources of many poor patient outcomes. Management, like medicine, is both art and science. Getting a handle on performance is the sine qua non of management. More specifically, to meet the exigencies of the science of management over the long haul, success depends on the valid measurement of performance and its components: quality, access, cost, and patient satisfaction. To improve performance, begin by improving management. To improve management, you need a yardstick—a means of comparing past with present and a way of determining how your organization stacks up against its peers, whether they are competitors or not. In short, you need a valid system of measuring performance.

In a sense, we are right back where we were—defining the characteristics or attributes of desirable performance measures. There is nothing mysterious or mystical in their definition. Such measures, as we discussed, must be reliable, valid, and useful. They are more likely to possess these attributes if they are based on healthcare events (processes or outcomes) that are frequent, as opposed to isolated. In addition, it is a real plus if the distribution of the events is approximately *normal* or bell-shaped.

The converse of the above axiom is: *You can't measure what you can't manage.* This axiom may not be as intuitively obvious as its counterpart, but it is just as important. *Measurement, or at least, scientific measurement (can it be otherwise), is almost impossible in an environment which is out of control, unmanaged, or unmanageable.* Scientific measurement *demands* a certain integrity of process incompatible with chaos. Chaotic environments are, in fact, not conducive to much of anything except further chaos.

The two axioms together illustrate what we mean by the *symbiosis of management and measurement.* We believe that good management and good measurement are equally important in contributing to organizational performance. We also believe that successful performance measurement systems must understand this symbiosis, at least intuitively, if they are to be successful. Like providers of care, performance measurement systems must be able to measure their own processes, outcomes, and linkages if they are to effectively manage their activities, such as the development of new performance measures. They must also be aware that they cannot reliably and validly measure their own activities and outputs if they cannot manage them. No matter what side of the fence one is on, management and measurement go hand-in-hand.

## ORGANIZATIONAL SYNERGY

When you have a well-managed healthcare organization really bent on improving performance, combined with a well-designed and responsive performance measurement system, you have the basis for synergetic outcomes. You also have a win-win situation, similar to that described by

Covey (1989): "With a Win/Win solution, all parties feel good about the decision and feel committed to the action plan . . . Win/Win is a belief in the Third Alternative. It's not your way or my way; it's a better way, a higher way" (p. 207). The bottom line is that cooperation between practitioners in healthcare organizations and those responsible for their performance measurement system, whether the latter is an internal or external party, is essential to this win-win situation.

# REFERENCES

1. Blum, M. L., and J. C. Naylor. 1968. *Industrial psychology: its theoretical and social foundations.* New York: Harper & Row.

2. Covey, S. R. 1989. *The seven habits of highly effective people: powerful lessons in personal change.* New York: Simon & Schuster.

3. Gillespie, R. 1993. *Manufacturing knowledge: a history of the Hawthorne experiments.* Cambridge: University Press.

4. Goonan, K. J. 1995. *The Juran Prescription: clinical quality measurement.* San Francisco: Jossey-Bass.

5. Hart, C. W. M. 1942. The Hawthorne experiments. *The Canadian Journal of Economics and Political Science.* 9:150–163.

6. Kazandjian, V. A., and T. R. Lied. 1998. Cesarean section rates: effects of participation in a performance measurement project. *Joint Commission Journal on Quality Improvement.* 6(4):201–204.

7. Rothlesberger, E. J., and W. J. Dixon. 1939. *Management and the worker.* Cambridge: Harvard University Press.

# CHAPTER

# 7

# Reports from the Field

*In the first six chapters of this book, we discussed factors related to the development and structure of performance measurement systems, including the actual humans involved in their conceptualization and implementation. With the possible exception of our discussion on the Hawthorne effect, we made little mention about the experiences of organizations that use these measurement systems. In chapter 7, we look at performance measurement systems within the context of real life organizations that have accepted their legitimacy, if not their absolute necessity to the organization's viability.*

*The characteristics and climate of an organization influence the choice of a performance measurement system within that organization. The organization is part of the economic, social, political, and healthcare structures and climate of a larger society—a society that will eventually pass judgment on the value of that organization via the marketplace or through that society's policing arm. Therefore, the vicissitudes of economic, social, and political forces will heavily influence the activities of an organization, including its selection of a performance measurement system.*

*We present four reports in which the issues of system design, evaluation, application, and* growing pains *are shared with the reader. The choice of field reports was intentional: we wanted to show how global the questions and the strategies that address these issues are. We offer the readers reports from Canada, the United States, and Australia that deal with unique aspects of the development and use of performance measurement systems in organizations that operate in somewhat diverse healthcare environments. We leave it to the reader to decide if these* case reports *provide evidence of successful implementation of the design and evaluation principles we have discussed so far.*

123

# REPORT #1

## THE ACHS CARE EVALUATION PROGRAM: A COMPREHENSIVE PROGRAM OF CLINICAL (MEDICAL) PERFORMANCE MEASURES

### *Joanne Williams and Brian Collopy*

Australia has a population of nearly 19 million served by approximately 1100 acute hospitals and 1500 long-term care facilities. Approximately 70 percent of the acute hospitals, with which this chapter is concerned, are public (government funded) and 30 percent private. There is a compulsory system of insurance (1.4 percent levy on income) called Medicare, which provides public hospital treatment and is free to pensioners and other welfare recipients. A decreasing proportion (now approximately 30 percent) of the population has additional private insurance enabling treatment in a private hospital or in a public hospital by the doctor of their choice. Specialist medical staff receive *fee for service* to private patients and generally in public hospitals are remunerated through a sessional or full-time salary. There are 10 medical schools which provide undergraduate education. Vocational training is conducted through the various medical colleges. There are approximately 50,000 medical practitioners, 40 percent of which are in specialist practice. Medical care in the larger public hospitals is provided by full-time medical staff in training and specialist medical staff, the majority of whom are *visiting* (sessional) medical officers. Smaller public hospitals, which are the majority, are served by visiting medical officers who may be specialists or general practitioners. Very few private hospitals have full-time *junior* medical staff.

The Australian Council on Healthcare Standards (ACHS) was established in 1974 along the lines of the Joint Commission in the United States to conduct organisation-wide accreditation surveys initially for acute healthcare organizations in Australia. Accreditation was conducted by surveyors (still actively employed in healthcare) visiting an organisation and viewing processes and documentation to determine whether or not given performance standards were being met. These standards were developed in consultation with the healthcare field and regularly updated in an Accreditation Guide. Critics of the accreditation process claimed it was bureaucratic and primarily focused on administrative issues. These early criticisms led to the introduction of concepts related to quality assurance to address clinical matters, and by 1983 the existence of a formal quality assurance program became a mandatory standard for accreditation. However, concerns continued to be expressed as to whether or not this standard had any impact on the quality of care. A survey of hospital QA programs in 1987 suggested that only 25 percent of such programs were effective.[1]

The incumbent chairman of the ACHS in 1985 was Mr Brian Collopy, a surgeon who had conducted surgical audits for many years. He began to explore the possible development of a national healthcare performance measurement system. From its inception this measurement system was perceived as educational, and therefore to involve the medical colleges, which are responsible for the standards of post-graduate medical education, was a logical step. Over four-year period discussions continued between the colleges and the ACHS, and in 1989 the Committee of Presidents of Medical Colleges committed its support of joint development of clinical indicators. During the same year the Federal government announced the allocation of 20 million dollars for a Case Mix Development Fund, and the ACHS maintained that the government should fund a program addressing quality if it was looking at cost containment. A grant of $80,000 was provided over a two-year period to establish what became known as the *Care Evaluation Program (CEP)*. Additional funds were provided by Baxter Pharmaceuticals at that stage to support the program, and it was envisaged that several sets of indicators would be developed over a three-year period. The program has been supported by successive Commonwealth Health Department grants since that time.

## INDICATOR DEVELOPMENT

A clinical indicator is defined as a *measure of the clinical management and outcome of care.* It is an objective measure of either the process or outcome of patient care in quantitative terms. Clinical indicators are not exact standards; rather, they are designed to be *flags,* which through collection and analysis of data can alert to possible problems and/or opportunities for improvement in patient care. There are three guidelines the CEP use as a basis for development for each set of indicators. These are that

- The data are available in healthcare organizations
- The indicator is relevant to clinical practice
- The measure is achievable

**Table 7.1.** Clinical indicator development activities.

| Stage | Activities | By Whom |
|---|---|---|
| 1) CI Drafting | • Formation of Working Party | College |
| | • Literature review | CEP |
| | • Development of draft clinical indicators | Working Party |
| | • Formatting of clinical indicators | CEP |
| | • Development of Results Book | CEP |
| 2) CI Testing | • Field Test Australia-wide. Min 10–15 sites | CEP/Test facilities |
| | • Results reported to CEP | Test facilities |
| | • Data analysis | CEP |
| | • Field Test Report developed | CEP |
| 3) CI Review & Publication | • Review of Field Test Report | Working Party |
| | • Clinical indicators revised | Working Party |
| | • Clinical indicators reformatted | CEP |
| | • College/Society approval | Working Party |
| | • Users' Manual and Results Booklet developed | CEP |
| | • Users' Manual and Results Booklet published and distributed | CEP/ACHS |
| 4) Incorporated into Accreditation | • Clinical indicators surveyed as part of Continuum of Care standard | ACHS |
| | • Data collected and submitted to CEP | Facilities |
| | • Aggregate data base developed | CEP |
| | • Facility and aggregate reports produced | CEP |

A protocol was devised for the development of each set of indicators and consists of four major stages with a number of subsidiary steps, as outlined in Table 7.1, from their drafting through to their introduction in the accreditation process.

The five steps involved in the drafting of the clinical indicators are self-explanatory. The working parties are formed from Fellows (members) nominated by the respective medical college as experts in the specific disciplines, and this has been one of the unique features of the CEP. Using clinicians whose expertise is recognised by their college has ensured college ownership of the clinical indicators. This official recognition has facilitated the broad acceptance of the indicators among clinicians. The development and formatting of draft indicators involves making sure that the indicators are phrased in such a way that there is no ambiguity and that definitions for all terms within the indicators are included.

Once the indicators have been drafted they are tested in clinical settings of various types (private/public, large/small) at between 10 to 15 sites throughout Australia. National testing is considered vital as the conditions (and resources) in healthcare organisations and the patient characteristics can vary considerably between different geographical locations around the country. A project officer visits each individual field test site prior to the commencement of data collection to provide instructions and answer any questions that the staff may have. Data collection methods are not prescribed, as part of the testing process is to determine how practical it is for different organisations to address the draft indicators. In the early stages of clinical indicator development, it was thought that testing for each set of indicators should undergo two stages, first field testing and then *pilot* testing within the accreditation process. However, experience showed that once the indicators were introduced into accreditation the hospitals addressed them, and testing within accreditation was unnecessary. Field test data are collected for a period of three months. In addition to recording the quantitative data needed for the indicators, qualitative information is also collected. This provides feedback on how the data have been collected and how easy or difficult it was to extract the information. Field test organisations have the opportunity to provide feedback on any aspect of the indicators and the data collection process. Once all the field test data have been collated and analysed, a report is written and distributed to the working party. The second phase of *pilot* testing, which was conducted for the first set of indicators, was extremely time-consuming and resource intensive for little return. It was decided that for subsequent indicator sets *beta* testing would occur in any case with the indicators in action, and they would undergo annual review to determine their acceptance and worth.

The working party reviews the initial field test report and revises the indicators where necessary. This may require reformatting of the indicators or more rigorous definitions. The revised indicators are then sent to the respective college for ratification before a Users' Manual is published

**Table 7.2.**   Standard format in which clinical indicators are presented.

| Indicator Topic | Missed Injuries (cervical spine) |
|---|---|
| **Rationale:** | Because of the potential catastrophic outcome of mishandling patients with cervical spine injury, it is essential that cervical spine injury be considered and excluded in all trauma patients on presentation. |
| **Definitions of Terms:** | • **Cervical spine injury** is defined as a fracture/subluxation or cervical cord injury.<br>• **Missed injury** occurs when a cervical spine injury is recorded as an inpatient discharge diagnosis, but not as an emergency department diagnosis. |
| **Type of Indicator:** | This is a comparative rate based indicator addressing the process of patient care. |
| **Indicator Data Format** | |
| **CI No. 1.2** *Numerator* | The total number of patients admitted via the emergency department with cervical spine injury not recorded as the emergency department diagnosis. |
| *Denominator* | The total number of patients admitted via the emergency department, with an inpatient discharge diagnosis of cervical spine injury, in the time period under study. |

and distributed to all member facilities of the ACHS accreditation program wishing to address the set. An example of a clinical indicator as it appears in a Users' Manual (Emergency Medicine) is shown in Table 7.2.

# THE ROLE OF CLINICAL INDICATORS IN ACCREDITATION

Since the introduction of a new accreditation process in January 1997, the Evaluation and Quality Improvement Program (EQuIP), the clinical indicators are surveyed as part of the accreditation process under the Continuum of Care standard. Initially they were reviewed as part of the hospital's medical quality assurance program. Healthcare organisations in EQuIP are

**Table 7.3.** Years in which clinical indicators were introduced for each specialty area.

| Year | Clinical Indicator Set | Number of Indicators |
|------|------------------------|----------------------|
| 1993 | Hospital-Wide Medical Indicators | 10 |
| 1995 | Obstetrics and Gynaecology | 20 |
| 1996 | Anaesthetics | 9 |
|      | Day Procedures | 5 |
|      | Emergency Medicine | 5 |
|      | Internal Medicine | 35 |
|      | Psychiatry | 29 |
| 1997 | Ophthalmology | 9 |
|      | Paediatrics | 8 |
|      | Radiology | 6 |
|      | Rehabilitation Medicine | 7 |
|      | Surgery | 53 |
| 1998 | Intensive Care | 5 |
|      | Dermatology | 19 |
|      | Pathology | 11 |

required to provide evidence of improving or moving toward improving performance by utilizing data. Organisations should use ACHS/College indicators to provide such data when relevant to the services they provide. If an organisation's results compare unfavourably with its peer group, it is expected to determine the reason and take action where appropriate; such actions would be demonstrated at the time of survey. However, none of the indicators are mandatory nor is compliance with a *threshold* (where established) for their peer groups. Organisations may also elect to develop their own indicators and demonstrate their usefulness at the time of survey. In such a situation, however, the CEP cannot provide comparative data.

Table 7.3 shows in which years each new set of indicators was introduced into the accreditation process and the number of indicators in each set in 1998. In the first three years of the program, organisations were required to submit clinical indicator data to the Care Evaluation Program (CEP) only during the years in which they were going for survey. Along with the introduction of EQuIP, which is based on continual improvement, came the facility for all members to submit data to the CEP and receive comparative reports every six months.

**Table 7.4.**    Number of organisations contributing data to the National
Aggregate Database.

| Year | Number of Sets Available | Number of Clinical Indicators | Organisations Submitting Data |
|------|--------------------------|-------------------------------|-------------------------------|
| 1993 | 1  | 15  | 115 |
| 1994 | 1  | 18  | 127 |
| 1995 | 2  | 34  | 188 |
| 1996 | 7  | 124 | 243 |
| 1997 | 12 | 208 | 513 |

# NATIONAL DATABASE

The data submitted to the CEP by individual organisations are confidential, and no data are released which could identify an individual facility. An annual report of the aggregate data is produced, which provides both quantitative and qualitative information about the indicators and the types of changes organisations have made as a result of indicator monitoring. The number of hospitals contributing data has increased each year as shown in Table 7.4.

# PROGRAM DEVELOPMENT ISSUES

The first college to participate in clinical indicator development was the Royal Australian College of Medical Administrators, and it accepted in good faith that what was developed was worthwhile. There were 15 clinical indicators in the first set, covering areas such as trauma, pulmonary embolism, hospital readmission, return to the operating room, hospital acquired infections, prescription medication and drug monitoring, and patient throughput. Although indicator areas were identified, it was not always easy to identify the relevant expert body for an area. For example, there was no apparent authority at that time to consult with on the development of clinical indicators for hospital acquired infection. Teaching hospital microbiologists were eventually identified as the most appropriate group for consultation in this area along with the Australian Infection Control Nurses Association.

Unforeseen problems also arose because of the progression of medical practice leading to rapid changes in recommendations. One of the original indicators required frequent monitoring of gentamicin serum levels at a time when gentamicin was administered according to an eight-hour regime. This indicator became problematic when it was recommended that gentamicin be administered only once in 24 hours.

Various other definitional issues have arisen with a number of the specific college indicators, and these are addressed at a yearly college working party review of the previous year's quantitative and qualitative data. At these annual reviews, conducted in June and July of each year, indicators may be added or deleted from a set, and definitions may be altered. Any changes are widely publicised and come into effect as of January in the following calendar year.

The development of the clinical indicator program as an enhancement to the established accreditation process may have initially been detrimental to the CEP. Many of the ACHS staff who were used to the standard survey process felt the clinical indicators were only a small part of the accreditation program, and therefore very little effort went into marketing the clinical indicators. Also, only one in ten of the hospital surveyors were clinicians, which may have restricted their understanding and appreciation of the value of the clinical indicator program. However, the hospitals were more accepting of the value of indicator monitoring, and as shown in Table 7.4, the number of organisations addressing clinical indicators has increased rapidly since the introduction of the CEP, and it fits well in the new process of EQuIP.

## PROGRAM GROWTH ISSUES

The rapid increase in the number of colleges participating, the number of indicators the colleges wished to develop, and the number of organisations contributing to the program caused an unexpected demand for improved computer technology. The original data were stored in dBASE files, but the CEP did not have a permanent staff member who had programming skills. As organisations began requesting feedback, it became necessary to reassess the current software and technology. In 1995 the database was rebuilt in Paradox and an automatic reporting ability was developed. Organisations which have not varied from the definitions given in the clinical indicator users' manuals are sent two comparative reports for each of the indicators they have addressed. The first report provides their own organisation's data and compares it with the aggregate data from all other organisations who contributed valid data for the same indicator. The second report compares their data with a peer group, which is determined from stratification variables. When organisations submit indicator data they are also asked to provide information on key variables within their facility which will allow all organisations which have contributed data to be stratified into groups. The stratification variables are determined by the working parties and vary depending on the particular set of indicators being addressed. Some indicator sets are stratified into groups based on the number of separations from the appropriate clinical unit, while others may be grouped according to a classification associated with the geographical location of the unit or the types of patient they accept. Organisations are also classified on whether they are privately or publicly funded.

A computerised results booklet (CRB) was introduced in 1997 to facilitate reporting, validation, and entry of data. This reporting tool is PC-based, and after completion of all necessary information, organisations download encrypted data to a computer disk and forward this to the CEP at the end of each reporting period. Consideration is now being given to the complex issues of computerised *data collection* systems to reduce the burden placed on healthcare organisations.

## RISK-ADJUSTMENT

The stratification variables also provide some limited risk-adjustment as size and type of facility reflect the case mix of a healthcare organisation.[2] The CEP receives no actual patient information to risk-adjust further, although some indicators are risk-adjusted in their format. For example, the indicator for coronary artery graft mortality rates has seven subsets for risk. It remains an issue for Hospital Wide indicators such as unplanned readmissions and hospital acquired bacteraemia, and a move to greater specificity with such indicators is being considered.

## HOSPITAL RESPONSES
## TO INDICATOR MONITORING

Along with the quantitative data, facilities report qualitative information on actions taken in response to indicator monitoring. In 1995, with only two sets of indicators in accreditation, they reported taking action on over five hundred occasions. A follow-up (by the CEP) of these actions has confirmed improvement in both patient management and outcome, for example, a reduction in complications such as nosocomial infection rates.[3]

In 1997, with 12 sets, approximately 4,500 actions were apparently induced by indicator monitoring. We believe as do Kazandjian et al.[4] that responsiveness is the best measure of the value of an indicator. The types of response noted by the CEP can be grouped as

- Improvement in the accuracy of in-hospital data collection
- Increase in quality improvement activities
- Revision of policies and procedures
- Further educational programs
- New staff positions
- Alteration to equipment

# FUTURE DIRECTIONS

## A Core Set of Validated Indicators

The CEP acknowledges the contribution of the medical colleges to the success of the program. It is because the colleges share ownership of the indicators that we have been able to progress to the point where half of the hospitals in the country contribute data to the CEP. However, because of the many interests of specific colleges, the program has expanded so that there are currently more than two hundred separate indicators covering 15 specialty areas. It is time to review and consolidate the number of indicators so that it is possible to provide the necessary support for organisations and ensure the value of the program. The resources of health care organisations are limited, and this restricts the number of clinical indicators they are able to address properly. We would prefer an organisation addressed a small number of indicators and used them to improve care than collect data for a larger number of indicators and be unable to act on their results. Attributes for a *core* set of indicators have been developed reflecting amongst other issues clinical importance, precision, resource intensity, their uptake, the size of the population impacted, and their responsiveness. It is intended, in relation to accreditation, to concentrate on such *core* indicators as they are identified over time in the yearly review process conducted by each working party on the previous year's qualitative and quantitative data.

## Indicators of Appropriateness

The two essential features of a healthcare service are that what is delivered is of a high quality and is appropriate to deliver. Just as the providers were the obvious group to determine standards of quality in care, so they are in relation to the appropriateness of care. It is thus an obvious extension of the CEP/college nexus to develop measures of appropriateness; for example, the justification for admission to hospital, the ordering of investigations, and the performance of procedures. Such a program would also provide a means of evaluating the level of adoption of, and adherence to, the numerous *best practice guidelines* which are being developed in Australia and many other countries and hailed as a means of reducing inappropriate care.[5] There is as yet limited evidence of their uptake and influence on care.[6]

## Multidisciplinary Measures

The CEP has been criticised for its *medical* practice concentration, which was a deliberate focus to increase medical staff involvement in *quality* activities.[7] However *system* problems are recognised as a frequent cause of adverse events in hospital,[8] and the CEP will move to involve nursing and other disciplines in the development of measures which involve other disciplines directly and which address the *continuum* of care.

## Consumer Involvement

While the CEP has intermittently consulted with consumer groups and recognised no inconsistency with consumer interest, there is a call to involve consumers on a more formal basis. The development of indicators in such areas as patient communication is contemplated.

## Benchmarking

The CEP publishes aggregate information on indicator rates stratified according to size, location (metropolitan or rural), and type (public or private).[9] In addition to this, both hospitals in EQuIP and those not in that program can utilise the services of the CEP and its national database to obtain information on their performance compared with a peer group.

## Link to Academic Research Units

As the indicators are being utilised more widely, the challenges to their validity and reliability have increased. In addition to the annual review and refinement of each indicator set, the CEP is being encouraged to establish formal ties to one or more recognised health research groups to increase the scientific *rigour* of the indicators used in its process of evaluation of standards in Australian acute healthcare.

# SUMMARY

The ACHS through the Care Evaluation Program was the first healthcare accrediting body to introduce clinical performance measures (indicators) into an accreditation program. With the cooperation of the medical colleges, a comprehensive group of indicators (over two hundred) have been successfully introduced over the five-year period from 1993.

Approximately half of the nation's acute hospitals (covering approximately 80 percent of the separations) address the indicators and forward quantitative and qualitative data. The responsiveness of the indicators is demonstrated by the large number of actions taken by hospitals, as a result of indicator monitoring, and reported to the CEP. There is ample documented evidence of improvement in patient management and outcomes.

The rapid growth in the program has increased the complexity of the CEP National database, which has been rebuilt to provide a computerised reporting system. Consideration is being given to computerised data collection systems for the organizations involved.

Despite refinement of the indicators through the ongoing (annual) review process for each set, challenges with regard to indicator validity continue. This is being addressed through the establishment of a *core* set of indicators which strongly comply with a number of generic and performance criteria. A further approach will be the linking of CEP with one or more research units to study areas with a limited *evidence base.*

A call to extend the indicator development to multidisciplinary measures and to ensure greater consumer involvement is being addressed. The CEP also has commenced to address the development of measures of *appropriateness* of care, which will encompass *best practice guidelines,* so that in addition to being able to determine that the care given was of a high quality there will be an assurance that it was justified.

# REFERENCES

1. Renwick, M., and R. Harvey. 1989. *Quality Assurance by hospitals: a digest.* Australian Institute of Health, Canberra.

2. Booth, J. L., and B. T. Collopy. 1997. *A National Clinical indicators database: issues of reliability and validity.* Australian Health Review. 20:84–95.

3. Portelli, R., J. Williams, and B. Collopy. 1997. Using clinical indicators to change clinical practice. *J. Qual. Clin. Practice.* 17:195–202.

4. Kazandjian, V., P. Wood, and J. Lawthers. 1995. Balancing science and practice in indicator development. *Int. J. Qual. Healthcare.* 7:39–46.

5. Woolf, S. H. 1990. Practice guidelines: a new reality in medicine. Recent developments. *Arch. Int. Med.* 150:1811–1818.

6. Schwartz, L. M., S. Waloshin, and H. G. Welch. 1996. Trends in diagnostic testing following a national guideline for evaluation of dyspepsia. *Arch. Int. Med.* 156:873–875.

7. Collopy, B. T., M. Z. Ansari, J. L. Booth, and J. A. Brosi. 1995. The Australian Council on Healthcare Standards Care Evaluation Program. *Med. J. Aust.* 163:477–80.

8. Leape, L. L., J. Lawthers, et al. 1993. Preventing medical injury. *Quality Review Bulletin.* 19:144–149.

9. Williams, J., J. Brosi, R. Portelli, et al. 1997. *Measurement of Care in Australian Hospitals.* Australian Council on Healthcare Standards.

# REPORT #2

## COLLABORATING TO IMPROVE CARE: A REGIONAL MODEL

*Rachel Rowe, R.N., M.S.*
*Michael Hill, M.Ed.*

Healthcare reform was a top priority for candidate Bill Clinton during his 1992 campaign for the presidency of the United States. After he took office, First Lady Hillary Clinton headed the effort to craft legislation aimed at changing the way healthcare in America is delivered and financed. While there was much controversy over the various proposals, expectations were high that some meaningful guidance for improving healthcare in the nation would result.

The national reform effort ended in 1994 when the U.S. Congress failed to pass the president's plan or any of the alternative proposals. As a consequence, reform would be market-driven, or a result of state or local, public or private initiatives. It was in that context that the New Hampshire Hospital Association (NHHA), a nonprofit hospital association, decided to proactively work to improve the healthcare delivery system statewide. Hospitals and physicians in this state had successfully worked together for many years on performance-related projects, so we approached this challenge optimistically.

NHHA invited the New Hampshire Medical Society to join us and engaged hospital administrators and physicians in attempting to answer the question, *What is good care, how do we measure it, and how do we make it better?* Regulatory and accrediting bodies had traditionally dictated how institutions should monitor performance. We felt that such a prescriptive approach, which would have been expanded under national legislation, inhibited the ability to assess the unique needs of our populations. It also hindered efforts to develop institutional and community-based strategies for improvement.

At the same time, there was growing interest in the potential for consumers to play a more significant role in changing the healthcare system. Two concepts evolved. Initially, policymakers focused on the concept that providing information to consumers would lead to better informed decision-making resulting in health system improvement. An alternative concept was patient-centered, involving the systematic collection of patient feedback and use of that information to target improvement efforts.

The approach popular among policymakers led to the publishing of *report cards* and rankings of hospitals and physicians. For several years in the 1980s, the federal government published hospital-specific mortality rates. Significant backlash from the provider and research communities about methodological flaws led the government to abandon this effort. Several years later, Pennsylvania and New York opted to publish hospital and physician-specific risk-adjusted mortality rates after coronary artery bypass surgery. Although mortality rates dropped 41 percent in the first four years following the release, debate continues as to the causative factors.

For example, could physicians be more carefully documenting coexisting conditions of their patients to improve their risk-adjusted rates? Or could publishing mortality rates by physicians influence their decisions about which patients are recommended for surgery (Blumenthal & Epstein, 1996)? These experiences indicate that more research is needed on how consumers make decisions about their care, what information is meaningful, and how that information should be presented (Cleary & Edgman-Levitan, 1997).

Given the uncertainty in the field about how to provide information to consumers that will be useful, we believed that the *patient-centered* approach would be the more powerful catalyst for change. Traditionally, information from medical records was the basis for evaluating and improving care. Patients' observations were not generally considered to be a useful tool in quality assurance activities. But experts in the field are beginning to recognize the value of patient feedback (Blumenthal, 1996). Patients are a source of important information about their treatment that is not available elsewhere.

We decided to pursue the *patient-centered* approach with two caveats. First, if patient feedback was to be used in the evaluation of performance and as a basis for change, it was critical that this feedback be collected by diagnosis. Only by asking questions related to the course of treatment and specific processes of care could physicians target their efforts at improving their practices and relating to patients. Second, the performance measurement system must capture the continuum of care. As hospital stays shorten and more care is delivered in physicians' offices or at home, it was critical to understand any opportunities for improvement in those settings. At this juncture, representatives from the Home Care Association of New Hampshire were invited to join the group.

# THE FOUNDATION FOR HEALTHY COMMUNITIES

How do you create a framework to facilitate efforts to improve diagnosis-specific care across the continuum over time? Could this be accomplished through the New Hampshire Hospital Association? Or was it necessary to create a new organization?

The Association's mission was to *improve health.* Despite being a *hospital* organization, we realized that involving only hospitals would limit our success. Hospitals were playing a less central role in the overall delivery of care than in the past, and we expected that trend to continue. Patients' experience in the delivery system prior to and after a hospital stay was becoming increasingly important. So our strategy for improving care would require us to broaden our focus beyond hospitals.

While hospitals in New Hampshire were our starting point, we would involve others who shared our goals. They would include executives and clinicians from organizations providing care outside the hospital, primary care physicians, and home care providers. Health insurance plans influence both the distribution of resources and the delivery of care so getting payers involved would be an important part of our strategy. It also made sense to expand beyond New Hampshire's borders by involving hospitals in neighboring states of Vermont and Maine. That would create a demographically larger database and more financial support.

But could NHHA serve as the base for getting a wide range of participants engaged in healthcare improvement initiatives? Probably not. Persuading essential players outside the Association's domain to commit resources, time, energy, and expertise to our vision would require a strong sense of partnership and ownership. The Association's 60-year history of serving only hospitals would likely be a handicap.

Some suggested that a foundation might be an effective model for pursuing collaborative quality and accountability initiatives involving many stakeholders. NHHA had a related education and research foundation in place, but it had no budget, no staff, and had been dormant for many years. Could a restructured Hospital Association Foundation serve as our bridge to the future? Might the new Foundation attract participation by potential partners who would be less inclined to link up with the Association directly? Probably. The Foundation concept made sense. It was the option NHHA decided to pursue.

This was our vision.

| Association | Foundation |
|---|---|
| With a community of interest focused on acute care | With a community of interest focused on improving health and healthcare delivery system-wide. |
| With interests neatly contained state within state boundaries | With interests overlapping boundaries |
| With hospitals as the exclusive members and participants | With membership and participation extended to hospitals, systems, health plans, and others who share our values and goals |

By September 1995, the mission, by-laws and name of our Hospital Association Foundation were revised. The notion of *healthy communities* summarized the stretching of boundaries beyond hospital care and coincided with language that hospitals were using to describe their own evolving sense of mission and heightened community focus. *Foundation for Healthy Communities* became the new name.

It is very difficult to secure support for a new venture. Previous efforts to establish an organization for pursuing quality improvement initiatives in New Hampshire had failed. Our strategy for dealing with the funding issues was not to count on finding new money to finance the Foundation, but rather to transfer existing staff and the funding to support them from the Hospital Association to the Foundation. The net financial effect was zero, given that the Association members viewed the Foundation as a sister enterprise, governed by the same group of trustees. So effective January 1, 1996, Association staff members engaged in information and quality activities, along with the financial support they needed, were formally transferred from the Association to the Foundation. The Foundation was up and running on the transfer date. One of the staff's first priorities would be to find ways to grow the Foundation by securing other sources of support. Shortly thereafter, the Medical Society and the Home Care Association offered additional financial support.

Our first round of projects was promoted as experiments. We told our member hospitals that we were looking for about six or eight hospitals to volunteer to participate. Twenty volunteered. Each participant was asked to contribute a small amount of money to supplement the transfer of money from the Hospital Association to the Foundation. Contributions ranged from $1500 for the smallest participant to $4000 for the largest.

In 1997, we were interested in encouraging all New Hampshire hospitals to participate. So we incorporated the cost of participation into every hospital's Hospital Association dues, with the amount to be transferred automatically to the Foundation. Support for the Foundation became an integral part of Hospital Association membership, and cost was eliminated as an issue in determining whether or not a member hospital would participate. In effect, they would be contributing to support Foundation projects whether they participate or not. We achieved 100 percent participation in 1997.

We saw health insurance plans as essential partners and potential lenders as well. Although the Association's track record of working with these groups was sporadic, an issue arose that provided a meaningful opportunity to encourage participation by plans.

In 1996 and 1997, health insurance plans were under fire in the U.S. Congress and in state legislatures because of an issue known as *drive through deliveries.* Plans were accused of forcing women out of hospitals too quickly after childbirth. It was suggested that plans were putting mothers and babies at risk in order to save money. The evidence was anecdotal. Nevertheless all plans, guilty or not, were caught up in a wave of unfavorable publicity regarding the care of mothers and newborns. Since the focus of our work in 1997 would be our *Maternal & Newborn Assessment Project,* we offered plans the opportunity to work with providers to assess and improve the care of mothers and newborns statewide and in the region. The plans were intrigued by a systematic, objective multistate initiative to measure patients' reports of care, especially relative to mothers and newborns. Eventually every plan doing business in New Hampshire would become partners in the Foundation.

With hospitals, health plans, physicians, and home care as partners, the Foundation for Healthy Communities had established its own center of gravity in sync with the Association. The Foundation uses the term *partner* to identify organizations that support the work of the Foundation financially. In 1997, the Maine Hospital Association joined as a partner and 12 Maine hospitals soon enrolled in the *Maternal & Newborn Assessment Project.* Several Vermont hospitals also joined. The Foundation became a truly regional entity.

# THE FOUNDATION'S WORK

In 1996, the Foundation partnered with The Picker Institute, a nationally recognized patient survey firm, to help design a system for soliciting patient feedback for use in targeting quality improvement efforts. Its goals were to

- Determine what aspects of care are most important to a select group of patients throughout the continuum of care
- Identify any variation in reported quality of care by patient
- Link patients' perceptions of care throughout the healthcare system
- Report this information to all providers of care
- Make changes that improve care

The approach was to use a reliable and valid survey tool to measure the aspects of performance that would meet the stated goals. We chose two populations to study: acute myocardial infarction (AMI) patients and mothers of newborns. These groups were selected because they had high patient volume and there was significant variation in length of stay and resource use.

For example, in 1996, patients suffering an AMI stayed an average of three days in some hospitals and six or seven days in others. Average costs for these hospitalizations ranged from $7500 to $20,000. These patients also had three potential modes of therapy, medical management, catheter-based interventions, or surgery. We were interested in understanding the differences in patient reports of care based on these three treatment modalities as well as how the processes differ between groups of patients undergoing the same intervention. Mothers delivering babies constitute the number one reason for admission to hospitals and have costs that vary by $2000 for an average two-day length of stay.

Patients were identified for the study in the hospital and were asked their permission to participate. Within a month after discharge, they were mailed comprehensive questionnaires covering seven dimensions of care including respect for patient preferences; coordination of care; information and education; physical comfort; emotional support; involvement of family and friends; and continuity and transition. These dimensions were identified using focus groups conducted by The Picker Institute and represent the most significant aspects of a patient's healthcare experience.

The surveys were carefully designed to focus on the experiences of the patient rather than on rating general aspects of their care. For example, rather than asking patients to rate *the courtesy of the staff* or *the efficiency of the admission process,* these questionnaires ask about specific actions taken by hospital staff that ought to have happened. This approach minimizes the potential for confounding factors such as patients' expectations, personal relationships, gratitude, or response tendencies related to gender, class, or ethnicity (Cleary et al., 1991). The survey instrument also covered questions developed by New Hampshire clinicians that were specific to the typical course of care for AMI and childbirth patients. This survey is shown in Table 7.5.

While we had high expectations for the value of this methodology, we worked hard to help all participants understand the value of the patient feedback. This was a challenge for some small and rural hospitals that only treated a few patients with these diagnoses. We emphasized the importance of the descriptive nature of the project rather than the statistical significance.

Another step we took to manage expectations was to conduct briefings for key legislators and public officials. Our goal was to inform them of the work of the Foundation and especially the *Maternal & Newborn Assessment Project.* This project related directly to their current legislative agenda regarding maternal length of stay. They were impressed that providers and health plans had come together voluntarily to address important quality of care issues. We promised to keep them informed as the projects evolved.

During 1997, over 1500 patients were asked about their experiences with the healthcare system following their heart attacks. Over 16,000 women, including every new mother in New Hampshire, were invited to provide feedback about their prenatal, childbirth, and postpartum experiences. Response rates were high for both groups at over 50 percent.

The results for both groups showed that patients had confidence in the doctors and nurses treating them. Patients also felt they were being treated with dignity and respect. However, the survey results showed that there was an opportunity to improve how providers educate patients about caring for themselves at home. Over 25 percent of AMI patients reported that they were not told about medication side effects to watch for at home or when they could resume usual activities. Over 25 percent of the mothers responded that they did not receive enough information about feeding or bathing their babies. This group also reported that they were not completely told what symptoms to watch for at home or when they could resume activities.

**Table 7.5.**   AMI and Maternal/Newborn Survey sample questions.

**Respect for Patient Preferences**

❏ Did you have enough say about your treatment?
❏ Did doctors (or midwives) talk in front of you as if you weren't there?

**Coordination of Care**

❏ Was there one particular doctor (or midwife) in charge of your care in the hospital?
❏ Were your scheduled tests and procedures performed on time?

**Information and Education**

❏ When you had important questions to ask a doctor (or a midwife), did you get answers you could understand?
❏ Did a doctor (midwife) or nurse explain the results of tests in a way you could understand?

**Physical Comfort**

❏ How many minutes after you pressed the call button did it usually take before you got the help you needed?
❏ Overall, how much pain medicine did you get?

**Emotional Support**

❏ Was it easy for you to find someone on the hospital staff to talk to about your concerns?
❏ Did you get as much help as you wanted from someone on the hospital staff in figuring out how to pay your hospital bill?

**Involvement of Family and Friends**

❏ Did your family or (someone close to you/birthing partner) have enough opportunity to talk to your doctor (or midwife)?

**Continuity and Transition**

❏ Did someone tell you about medication side effects to watch out for when you went home?
❏ Did someone on the hospital staff tell you what danger signals (about your illness or operation/in you and your baby) to watch out for when you went home?

*Source:* © The Picker Institute, Boston, MA. 1995. Developed in collaboration with the Foundation for Healthy Communities, Concord, New Hampshire

Understanding what patients think about their healthcare experience is meaningful only if that information can be used to create change in the processes that will lead to an improved delivery system (Batalden & Stolz, 1993). The Foundation for Healthy Communities developed an approach to help make that happen. There were several steps in this process.

Concurrent with the surveys, the Foundation worked with researchers from Dartmouth Medical School to document the processes of care that these patients go through from prehospital care through their transition home. The goal was to understand what the processes were and what made them good or bad from the perspective of both the patients and the clinicians. To accomplish this, the Foundation conducted focus groups in small, medium, and large hospitals throughout New Hampshire. Our objective was to assess real or perceived differences based on demographics, provider mix, or availability of resources.

The focus groups revealed several significant differences with the *qualitative* aspects of the processes rather than the processes themselves. For example, mothers from small and rural hospitals valued staying in their community with providers they knew and trusted and having family support nearby. Mothers from large hospitals were more concerned about the relationship with their physician and the amount of information they received from their clinicians. These qualitative aspects were identified as potential contributors to differences in patient care. A map was created from the focus group feedback that documents the processes of care throughout the continuum.

The next step was to connect the survey questions to the processes on the map. This would allow hospitals and physicians to review their results and identify the steps in the processes of care that likely contribute to the patients' perceptions. For example, they could answer questions such as: *At what point in the process should an AMI patient learn about the side effects of his medications?* From this information, clinicians could focus on immediate next steps and target change efforts.

This linkage also allowed for benchmarking. The Foundation's strategy was to use the survey results to identify hospitals that have processes in place that correlate with the most favorable feedback from AMI and maternity patients. We encouraged the formation of process improvement teams within and between hospitals. These teams continue to work individually and collaboratively to learn from the experience of those providers who are achieving the best results.

# SUCCESSES AND FUTURE CHALLENGES

The ultimate measure of success for the Foundation is the extent to which we play a role in actually improving health and healthcare. For example, we now have baseline data on the care of mothers and newborns and strategies for helping clinicians in the field effect change. The data we collect a year or two from now will give us some tangible indication of whether or not our work appeared to make a difference.

In the interim, we accept as an indicator of success that many clinicians and administrators are enthusiastically embracing the Foundation for Healthy Communities' initiatives. The survey results reveal both the strengths and the weaknesses in their clinical programs and administrative systems. The process maps produced through the Foundation are helping them focus on specific aspects of care that may need change.

The health insurance plans also continue to support the Foundation. They are using their member-specific data to evaluate the effectiveness of their prenatal care and cardiac rehabilitation programs.

The Foundation attributes its success largely to

- A *patient-centered* philosophy in improvement efforts
- Participation is voluntary
- An environment that fosters adaptability, creativity, and change
- A regional approach to improving the healthcare delivery system
- An approach that emphasizes guiding principles rather than a grand design

Despite the success of the Foundation, we have many challenges that lie ahead if we are to measurably improve care to patients. These include

- Educating the chief executive and trustee leadership about the importance of using patient feedback and process knowledge to reduce variation and improve care in their institutions

For example, we established an annual Invitational Summit Conference on Improvement for hospital CEOs, trustee leaders, medical staff leaders, and nurse executives. We are also diligent about providing positive feedback about their organization's participation and the outstanding efforts of the staff who are directly involved in our work on a day-to-day basis.

- Demonstrating that improving care can enhance the competitiveness and future viability of providers and plans

National experts are working with us to share information about how performance information is increasingly being used by purchasers, including business coalitions and government programs, to evaluate the overall cost-effectiveness of providers and health plans.

- Financing the continuing collection of patient data to monitor the effectiveness of interventions and to promote process improvement on a continuous basis

We are considering more cost-effective methods of maintaining our databases including sampling techniques and finding new sources of financial support.

- Discouraging the use of patient feedback for marketing purposes

We are constantly emphasizing that our goal is improve care system-wide, and that collaboration rather than competition is the key to accomplishing that.

- Educating purchasers, policymakers, the media, and consumers about how information about patient feedback and the process knowledge is being used to improve care

Efforts in this regard have included special presentations before public officials, news releases describing our work, radio advertising, and press releases.

- Discovering ways of sharing data with purchasers, policymakers, the media, and consumers as a means of facilitating more informed decisions about healthcare policy and decision making

While the purpose of our work is to improve health and healthcare, we are also attempting to learn from the experience of others who have made data public for the expressed purpose of helping consumers make decisions. Unfortunately there are few examples of success in this regard. This is a challenge that we'll continue to explore.

Since its inception in 1995, The Foundation for Healthy Communities has proved to be an effective facilitator for healthcare improvement efforts in New Hampshire and Northern New England. The participants have a genuine sense of ownership. The Foundation has become a *white space* for pioneering efforts in using patient feedback and process knowledge to improve the healthcare delivery system.

# REFERENCES

1. Batalden, P. B., and P.K. Stoltz. 1993. A framework for the continual improvement of health care: building and applying professional and improvement knowledge to test changes in daily work. *The Joint Commission Journal on Quality Improvement.* 19(10):424–452.

2. Blumenthal, D., and S. M. Epstein. 1996. The role of physicians in the future of quality management. *The New England Journal of Medicine.* 335(17):1328–1331.

3. Cleary, P. D., and S. Edgman-Levitan. 1997. Health care quality: incorporating consumer perspectives. *Journal of the American Medical Association.* 278(19):1608–1611.

4. Cleary, P. D., S. Edgman-Levitan, M. Roberts, et al. Winter 1991. Patients evaluate their hospital care: a national survey. *Health Affairs.* 254–267.

# REPORT #3

## Supporting the Use of Data for Improvement: Lessons Learned from a National Pilot Test in Canada

*Nancy Gault*
*Nancy Kelly*
*Cathy Davis*
*Regina Coady*
*Mark Mycyk*

In 1994, the Canadian Council on Health Services Accreditation (CCHSA), in collaboration with the Canadian Institute for Health Information (CIHI), initiated its Performance Indicators Project.[1] The first phase of the project began with selecting and pilot testing six performance indicators generic to acute care services. As the pilot test nears completion, the results of the pilot test have been instructive in many ways to those of us who participated in its implementation and evaluation.

*What we did not know, going into the pilot test, was the absolute importance of building good process. In other words, using indicators is not just about data and reports; supporting the user in understanding the data and translating that understanding into improvement requires constant communication, education, and other financial and human resources. Over the course of the project, we have learned as much about the structures and processes required to support indicator usage as we have learned about the reliability and usefulness of the six indicators being pilot tested. In this chapter, we will share what we have learned through the pilot test.*

## THE CANADIAN CONTEXT

*In Canada, the responsibility for health services falls predominantly under provincial jurisdiction. Despite this, the federal government has wielded considerable influence over the delivery of health service by providing*

---

[1]CCHSA, in existence since 1958, is a national, nongovernmental agency that delivers accreditation programs for comprehensive health systems, acute care, cancer, long-term care, rehabilitation, mental health, home care and community health service organizations in Canada. Approximately 1500 organizations are accredited by CCHSA on a voluntary basis.

*funding to the provinces for health services (Sutherland & Fulton, 1988). Over the last decade, federal funding transfers to each of the provinces have decreased by varying amounts (Caragata, 1998). Faced with increasingly difficult financial restraints, many provincial governments initiated significant restructuring and downsizing of their healthcare systems.*

*Within this environment of cost containment and rapid system restructuring, many stakeholders, including the general public and healthcare providers, began expressing concerns about the quality of health services and access to services. Consequently, all stakeholders began demanding more information about the performance of health service organizations and the impact of ongoing changes on the quality of care and service.*

In response to this increasing pressure for accountability, government, insurers, and healthcare providers became interested in the development and use of indicators as a tool or mechanism for evaluating and monitoring the quality of care and service. As interest in performance measurement and the use of indicators took hold in healthcare, CCHSA had already initiated a major revision of the accreditation program. This revision resulted in the introduction of the Client Centred Accreditation Program (CCAP) in 1995 and set the stage for introducing the concept of performance indicators into the accreditation program. In the revised program, teams were required to select and monitor performance indicators relevant to their specific areas and report on them at the time of the accreditation survey.

*At the same time that CCAP was taking shape, members of CCHSA's Board of Directors and a group of interested surveyors had also begun discussions about the feasibility of identifying a core set of national performance indicators. The impetus for these discussions had come from a briefing paper written by a member organization. This small group of interested parties grew into a national steering committee with representation from the Canadian Hospital Association, the Canadian Institute for Health Information, research institutes, and healthcare organizations. From there grew the Performance Indicators Project.*

The goal for the project is to identify a common list of indicators that, in conjunction with the accreditation standards, can be used to support health services organizations in quality monitoring and improvement activities. By achieving a national consensus on a common set of indicators, CCHSA aims to facilitate the exchange of comparable data across Canada, and promote benchmarking across accredited organizations. This consensus building will take place over several years and will involve extensive field consultation and the use of expert technical committees.

Because CCHSA's standards cover all aspects of organizational performance, indictors will be developed for all levels of care and service including clinical areas, governance and management functions and support areas such as human resource management. Subsequent to pilot testing, the indicators developed through the project will be published with the accreditation standards. For the foreseeable future, their use by accredited organizations will be a voluntary component of the accreditation program. Over time, the ultimate test of the acceptability of the indicators will be the extent to which organizations across Canada actually use the indicators for quality monitoring and improvement.

## CCHSA'S APPROACH TO INDICATOR USE

*In addition to identifying and testing performance indicators, the steering committee saw the project focusing on education and on helping organizations to use indicators for quality improvement. From the beginning, the project has supported the use of indicators within the larger framework of quality improvement. Indicators are seen as a tool or guide to monitor, evaluate, and improve the quality of patient/client care, support services, and organizational functions that affect patient/client outcomes. Indicators* flag *when there are potential problems in quality. An in-depth analysis by the team or users is essential to determine whether there is, in fact, a quality of care or service issue to be addressed.*

*CCHSA believes that a judgment about the quality of care and service cannot be made in isolation of this detailed analysis. As such, CCHSA's focus is not so much on the indicator results themselves (for example, the numbers) as it is on the team's use of the information to evaluate and improve their processes of care and client outcomes.*

## PARTNERING WITH THE CANADIAN INSTITUTE FOR HEALTH INFORMATION

*CCHSA recognized, from the beginning, the importance of establishing a collaborative partnership with the Canadian Institute for Health Information (CIHI). CCHSA never saw itself as the collector of indicator data given CIHI's role and expertise in this area. Similar to CCHSA, CIHI is a private, not-for-profit organization with the mandate to coordinate the development and maintenance of a comprehensive and integrated health information system for Canada. It plays a key role in developing standards for health information, maintaining a number of national health databases, and providing value-added resource utilization information through national comparative reporting.*

## CCHSA'S INDICATOR DEVELOPMENT PROCESS

The Performance Indicators Project was set up to proceed in three phases. As with any large undertaking, it is often better to begin with something fairly targeted and manageable. Hence, Phase I of the project started with identifying and developing six indicators for one healthcare sector only—the acute care sector. Phase I was seen as an opportunity to gain some experience in indicator work, to get a feel for the resources required to support such work, and to determine the feasibility of indicator development on a larger scale. Figure 7.1 shows the phases of the Performance Indicators Project.

## SELECTING THE SIX ACUTE CARE INDICATORS

*Selection of the six indicators for Phase I was not as simple or straightforward as might have been expected. The task for selecting the indicators fell to a newly formed technical committee, which met four times over a period of a year and a half. The steering committee had established the following parameters for selecting the indictors for Phase I.*

- The focus for Phase I would be on *generic* indicators that could be applied to and reported by all care groups

- The rationale for each indicator would be based on one of the seven dimensions of quality used in CCSHA's standards— acceptability, effectiveness, appropriateness, efficiency, accessibility, safety, and competence

- The indicators would be based on data, which were available within organizations and were already submitted to CIHI

*It took a number of false starts before the committee was comfortable with a process for selecting the indicators. Eventually, the selection of the indicators became an iterative process in which a long list of indicators was gradually reduced as it went from the technical committee to the advi-*

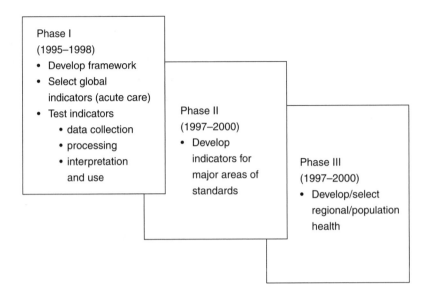

**Figure 7.1.** Phases of the Performance Indicators Project.

*sory committee and back again. Given that CIHI's hospital databases have historically collected data related to utilization, the final selection of indicators reflected a focus on utilization and the appropriateness of care.*

The final list of indicators was approved early in 1996 and consisted of the following indicators

1. Percentage of alternate level of care days (ALC)

$$\% \text{ ALC days} = \frac{\text{sum of ALC length of stay (LOS)} \text{ for all cases with an ALC LOS}}{\text{total LOS for an inpatient (acute setting) cases}}$$

A patient is considered ALC when he/she does not require acute care treatment, but occupies an acute care bed, usually awaiting placement in a chronic unit, home for the aged, nursing home, rehabilitation facility, other extended care institution, or home care program. The indicator supports the review of discharge planning, by assessing the degree to which patients have timely access to continuing care services.

2. Percentage of cases classified as May Not Require Hospitalization (MNRH)

$$\%\text{MNRH cases} = \frac{\text{total impatient (acute) cases with a}}{\text{total inpatient (acute) cases}}$$

The purpose of this indicator is to flag diagnoses where treatment may be given in an ambulatory setting. Case mix groups (CMGs) designated as MNRH are based on statistical information, inpatient length of stay, the percentage of hospital cases treated as same-day surgery and clinical judgment. This indicator supports the review of admissions to identify utilization management opportunities.

   3. Percentage of unplanned readmissions to the same hospital with the same or related diagnosis within 7 days of discharge

$$\%\text{ unplanned readmissions} = \frac{\text{the count of cases coded as an unplanned readmission}}{\text{count of total inpatient (acute setting) hospital cases}}$$

*The purpose of this indicator is to distinguish between readmissions to hospital within one week which are planned as part of the regular course of treatment and those readmissions resulting from complications or an adverse occurrence related to a previous inpatient admission. The indicator supports an assessment of the safety of discharge planning and the effectiveness of the community supports and services, which provide assistance to patients once they are discharged.*

*The readmission code is a one-digit code which is used to show a readmission to the same level of care within the reporting facility with a same or related diagnosis and which is judged to be unplanned.*

A *same or related diagnosis* refers to a presenting complaint which is the same or may be a symptom of the diagnosis from the previous admission and/or a presenting complaint occurring in the same body system, excluding obvious external causes or conditions obviously resolved in the previous admission and/or a stated complication or exacerbation related to the diagnosis from the previous admission.

An *unplanned readmission* is an unexpected or unanticipated inpatient readmission. A health records coder will make the judgment based on the patient's written history, mode of entry, and admission code.

   4. Percentage of cases which are day surgery

$$\% \text{ cases which are DS} = \frac{\text{count of surgical DS cases}}{\text{count of surgical DS and surgical inpatient (acute) cases}}$$

*The indicator supports the review of the appropriateness of the surgical cases provided in an ambulatory care setting. This review may also consider community services available to support post–surgical patients in the community following a day procedure. DS procedures generally require the use of an operating room suite and a post–anaesthesia or post–recovery room for patients who do not need to be admitted to an inpatient bed and who are discharged within 24 hours following surgery.*

5. Percent of days over/under expected length of stay (LOS)

$$\frac{\% \text{ days over / under}}{\text{expected LOS}} = \frac{\text{sum of total length of stay} - \text{the sum of the expected length of stay}}{\text{the sum of the expected length of stay}}$$

The expected length of stay (LOS) is based on *typical* cases calculated by one of five potential models developed by CIHI. The organization's LOS is compared to the expected LOS by the number and/or percent of days greater than or less than the expected LOS. The indicator supports the review of LOS outliers as part of a measure of the efficiency of inpatient resources.

6. Average length of stay in the emergency department for patients designated as admitted to the organization

$$\frac{\text{Average LOS in ER}}{\text{for admitted patients}} = \frac{\text{sum of (time of discharge from ER – admission time) for all patients admitted form ER}}{\text{total number of patients admitted from ER}}$$

*This indicator measures the length of stay from the time the patient is designated as admitted until the patient is transferred to the inpatient unit for all patients admitted to the organization through the Emergency Department (ER). The indicator supports the review of efficiencies related to the admission process from ER.*

## PURPOSE OF THE PILOT TEST

*Having selected the list of indicators, the steering committee outlined the following questions to be addressed by the pilot test.*

What are the reliability issues related to each indicator?

Was the indicator information useful in supporting decision making?

Did the indicators help the organization to improve the quality
of care and service provided?

What factors support the use of performance indicators?

# SETTING UP THE PILOT TEST

*Sixteen sites, with representation from each of the ten provinces, were chosen to participate in the pilot test. The organizations ranged from small organizations with under 50 beds to large, multisite, teaching organizations and were selected only if they had already undergone an accreditation survey under the Client-Centred Accreditation Program (CCAP). It was important for participating organizations to have demonstrated a commitment to performance measurement and the principles of quality improvement which underlie CCAP.*

For indicator use to be successful, it needs to be integrated into an organization's ongoing activities and structures (Angaran, 1991). Therefore, CCHSA's staff visited each of the pilot sites to meet with the organization's senior management and discuss how they saw the project fitting with their own goals and performance measurement initiatives. An exception to this was six organizations that joined as the Toronto Academic Health Science Council (TAHSC) that were treated as a single site. The lack of face-to-face contact with these six organizations' senior management and staff resulted in difficulties later in the project. These difficulties related to their partial understanding of their role in the project and the commitment required for the data collection and team analysis.

To give the pilot test some exposure within the organizations, CCHSA staff and the pilot site coordinators also met with team leaders, staff, physician groups, and health records staff. In many cases, these meetings helped to identify and resolve issues and concerns about implementing the project within the organizations.

## Identifying Users of the Indicator Reports

Organizations were asked to identify which of their teams would be looking at the reports for each of the six indicators. In a similar project, Barnsley et al. (1996) had stated the importance of identifying end users and developing a dissemination plan up front. The focus on teams stemmed from the philosophy underlying CCAP that staff involved in delivering care and service should also be involved in evaluating and improving the quality of care and services. As such, organizations were encouraged to identify direct care provider teams rather than management teams.

In actuality, many of the indicator reports ended up being used by coordinating and utilization committees rather than clinical teams. This is consistent with the findings of Barnsley et al. (1996) who identified a *clinical* versus a *system* perspective in their study. From a clinical perspective, direct care providers may be more interested in diagnosis-specific or procedure-specific outcome indicators than in the more global indicators that focus on resource allocation or management procedures. Therefore, when identifying the most appropriate user of the indicator information it is important to identify the purpose of the indicator. Indicators are used for different purposes throughout the organizations whether it is at a corporate level for resource management or at a clinical level for process improvement related to clinical activities.

Use of the indicator data also depends on how decision making is carried out in the organization. CCHSA encourages organizations to involve direct care and service providers in decision making. This represents a cultural shift for many organizations. Although all of the organizations in the pilot test had developed team structures within their organization, using indicator data and doing analysis at the team level would be a new activity for many of them. Later evaluations showed that this might not be a realistic expectation for some organizations at this time.

## DATA COLLECTION AND REPORTING

Beginning in October 1996, data for the six indicators were submitted to CIHI's discharge abstract databank (DAD), which is one of the most comprehensive national databases of its kind. Organizations across Canada abstract and submit patient-specific data including both clinical and demographic data elements to the DAD.

*To maintain data quality, CIHI has an extensive system of data edits to process discharge abstract data. Additional edits were added to this system to ensure that the data would conform to the data collection protocol. For example, for every readmission, health records staff were required to code whether the readmission was planned or unplanned. CIHI's editing system produced error messages to organizations when invalid, suspect or missing data were encountered. Pilot organizations were given two weeks to submit corrections for these error conditions.*

Approximately six to eight weeks after data submission, CIHI produced quarterly comparative indicator reports. These reports graphically displayed the indicator rates calculated from the DAD. Each indicator was then broken down and reported by different categories including case mix group (CMG)[2], doctor service, patient age, and so on. Sites were also given the edited data on a diskette from which they were able to produce their own customized reports and to *drill* down the data for more specific comparisons. Unlike similar indicator projects, the indicator data were not confidential; the data from all of the sites were made available to all participating organizations in both the reports and the diskette.

*Organizations were required to submit their abstract information to CIHI within 45 days—shorter than the 60 days normally required by CIHI. For some organizations, this was a significant shift in their current practice and in a few cases resulted in extra staff being brought in to support the pilot test. In some organizations it was clear that senior management, in committing to the project, had not fully understood the repercussions to the health records staff of committing to a 45-day submission cut-off. The resulting frustration of the health records staff became apparent when discussions around reliability issues began.*

## ASSESSING RELIABILITY AND DATA QUALITY

The first purpose of the pilot test was to identify reliability issues related to the indicators. Reliability was defined as the accuracy and consistency of the documentation, and of the abstraction and coding of the data elements. CCHSA identified a number of specific questions to be answered through the pilot test.

| Question | Mechanism for Assessment |
|---|---|
| How consistently is indicator information documented on the patient record? | → • identification of processes used to document indicator information |
| How consistently is the information abstracted and coded? | → • data quality surveys<br>• CIHI data edits |

---

[2]Case mix group is a registered trademark of CIHI.

To answer these questions, CCHSA and the pilot site staff first had to identify the processes used by care and service providers to document the data elements. During the initial site visit, CCHSA staff met with health-care providers and health records staff to ensure that everyone had the same understanding of the data collection methodology. This proved to be valuable in that it highlighted where efforts were needed to standardize mechanisms for documentation within a site and across sites.

*Once data collection began, a series of teleconferences were held with pilot site coordinators, health records staff, and CIHI to further identify inconsistencies in data collection and to discuss common issues and solutions for improving documentation.*

*For example, with the alternate level of care indicator (ALC) some organizations had developed a form for the physician or discharge planner to fill out when the patient no longer needed acute care services. This form was shared with the other organizations. Compliance with documentation was also an issue, especially for the ER indicator where the rate of documentation ranged from 33 percent to 98 percent.*

*Health records staff were asked to identify specific areas where there was potential for variation in the abstraction and coding of specific data elements. CCHSA subsequently developed data quality surveys in which health records staff were given a series of different scenarios and were asked how they would code the data elements. Data quality surveys were considered a low cost alternative to reabstractions studies, which were not feasible given the geographical spread of the pilot sites and limited resources. Despite this, the data quality surveys did demonstrate some disconcerting results. For example, in a recent data quality survey, health records staff was given a series of scenarios relating to unplanned readmissions. Staff were asked to identify whether the readmission was planned or unplanned. In one scenario, 37 percent of staff coded the readmission as planned and 63 percent of staff coded it as unplanned.*

*At the beginning of the project, it was thought that the teams would be able to use the data as soon as they received the first comparative report. Instead, the first year of the pilot was spent discussing and then making changes to indicator definitions to improve the consistency of coding. Obviously, achieving data quality is an evolving step by step process that takes time. It is hard to get good data at the outset. In fact, it seems that data quality only becomes important when the users start to look the data. Pink et al. (1998) stated that "bad data are often hard to detect and sometimes not revealed until used in a performance comparison." Yet, better quality data doesn't come without effort—achieving good quality data means organizations must have the methods and tools (and perseverance) in place for assessing and then improving data quality on an ongoing basis.*

### Comparability of the Indictor Data

*One of the challenges of working across different provincial jurisdictions is to achieve a common understanding and agreement about the data elements. Comparing indicator data across provinces has been always been hindered by the fact that the provinces have historically developed different definitions for the same indicators. Furthermore, provinces have different funding formulas, which in some cases influenced how the data elements were documented. For example, with the alternate level of care (ALC) indicator, some provinces have financial incentives to document ALC accurately, while other provinces apply financial penalties to the patient which makes physicians reluctant to designate a patient as ALC. The comparability issues raised by system differences such as these go beyond the scope of this pilot test.*

There was no doubt that the pilot organizations were well aware of these comparability issues. They needed to feel comfortable that they were comparing themselves to organizations that were similar to theirs. Therefore, based on their suggestions, profile information on each of the sites was collected and then shared among the sites. For example, large teaching hospitals with tertiary cardiac services wanted to compare themselves to other hospitals with the same type of services. These types of comparisons were somewhat limited due to the small sample size of the pilot.

*The pilot test demonstrated that assessing and evaluating reliability probably takes six months to a year when there are multiple organizations involved and comparability across organizations is an issue.*

## ASSESSING USEFULNESS OF THE INDICATORS

*The second purpose of the pilot test was to answer two questions about the usefulness of the indicators. In other words, was the indicator information useful in supporting decision making and did the indicators help the organization to improve the quality of care and service provided? In its initial discussions, the steering committee decided to avoid using the term validity as they felt it would create confusion among participants. Usefulness, on the other hand, is a fairly concrete term that has meaning to most people.*

*The tool for evaluating usefulness was a team questionnaire. CCHSA sent this questionnaire to participating teams at various times throughout the pilot test to track indicator usage over the duration of the pilot test. The questionnaire focussed on the teams' perceptions of the indicators and asked them to document any changes they had initiated based on the indicator data.*

*The survey questions focused on five sequential stages of indicator use based on the Maryland Hospital Association's (1993) 5 W's of quality management and stages of decision theory. By asking a series of questions related to each of the levels, we were able to ascertain, for each indicator, the level of use by the teams. The following is a description of the framework used for the questionnaire.*

| Level of Usage | Project Framework | 5 W's |
|:---:|---|---|
| 1 | Did the team look at the indicator data? | Where am I? |
| 2 | Did the team further investigate or look for more information based on the indicator data? | Why am I here? |
| 3 | Did the team determine that there were opportunities for improvement based on where they wanted to be? | Where do I want to go? |
| 4 | Did the team initiate any changes? | What will I do? |
| 5 | Did the team use the indicator reports to monitor change and were there improvements? | What did I accomplish? |

*The first questionnaire was sent to 59 teams involved in the pilot test after they had received the fourth comparative indicator report from CIHI. Given the emphasis that had been placed on teams, it was surprising to find that in many cases, the indicator reports had not made it past the team leaders. Therefore, one of the first lessons was the importance of ensuring reports reached team members. These reports are shown in Figures 7.2–7.5.*

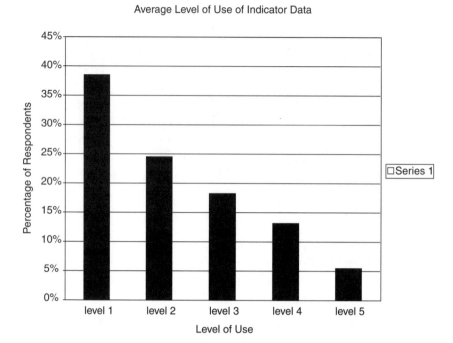

**Figure 7.2.**   Level of indicator use by indicator.

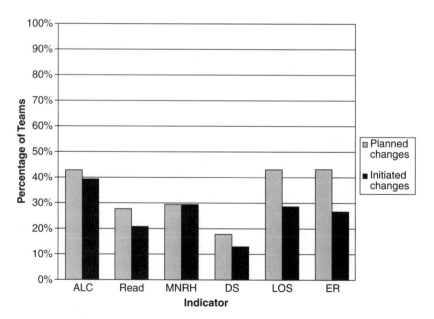

**Figure 7.3.**   Percentage of teams monitoring indicator that planned and
initiated change to processes.

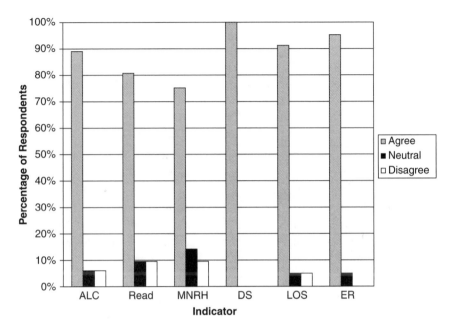

**Figure 7.4.**   Relevance of indicators to the team's work.

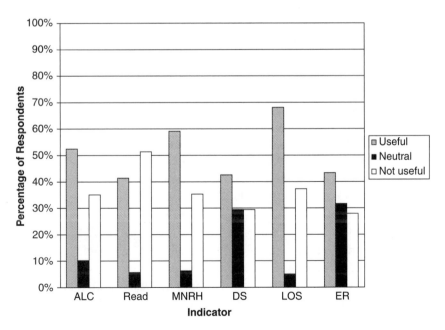

**Figure 7.5.**   Usefulness of indicators in identifying opportunities for improvement.

*The actual survey results were not surprising; many of the teams had reached level 1 in usage (for example, where am I?). A smaller percentage of the teams had reached the level where changes were actually undertaken and then monitored (level 5). The following is a graphic display of the level of indicator usage by the teams based on the levels described above and the percentage of teams that actually implemented changes.*

There may be many reasons for these results. An initial thought was tha the cycle for process improvement might take longer than what was provided. As the survey is repeated over time, the levels of usage may increase just because teams will have had more time to plan for and implement change. Ownership was another issue that the teams identified as a factor affecting usefulness. Although the teams received the reports, in some cases the factors or processes that affected the indicator rates were not under their control. For example, the rate for alternate level of care days is influenced by the availability of long-term care beds in the community.

Another factor that may have influenced the results is the team members' degree of skills or knowledge. Some team members, in response to the questionnaire, stated that they did not know how to read or interpret the indicator reports. This point was further illustrated by the fact that although approximately 80 percent of the teams said that the indicators were relevant to their work, when asked about the usefulness of the indicators in helping them to identify opportunities for improvement, fewer teams agreed with the statement.

A number of the pilot organizations said that they were unable to support data usage at the team level. Usually the smaller community organizations did not always have the information systems in place to support *drilling* down of the data to a level that was meaningful to the team. In other cases, organizations did not have sufficient health records staff to help team members interpret the reports. Although a guide was produced to explain the reports, many team members needed more support to understanding the process of coding and how data elements get translated into the calculation of the indicator rates.

Another factor affecting indicator use was the organizations' level of functioning and previous experience. Some of the organizations had already done significant analysis and process improvement around the pilot test indicators. These organizations were less likely to say that the indicator data from the pilot had prompted them to change. The pilot sites also said that they do not always initiate change based on one indicator; teams may use a collection of three or four indicators to build an accurate picture of their care and service. Yet, the evaluation questionnaire had specifically asked teams to evaluate the indicator in isolation of other indicators.

Finally, many of the pilot organizations are still undergoing significant change within their organizations due to system restructuring. There is the real possibility that the pressures of other projects took precedence over this pilot test. Thus, establishing the usefulness of indicators is a complex process. It is difficult to separate and then evaluate all of the different factors that affect whether an organization will use indicator information. A question not yet answered is, how long does it take to evaluate the usefulness of an indicator? It may be that it takes a two-year period to comfortably determine whether an indicator is useful in making improvement.

## VALUE OF PARTICIPATING IN THE PROJECT

Throughout the pilot testing, organizations reported many positive benefits from participating in the pilot test. The most important was that the pilot test raised team members' level of awareness about indicators and their use. They gained an understanding of how indicator data could be used to support decision making. Giving staff comparative data provided a focal point for them to discuss and evaluate their processes in a learning environment. Team members also became sensitive to the importance of good data and good documentation. The role of coding and the health records function was more clearly understood and this mutual understanding helped providers and health records staff work collaboratively to achieve team goals.

Another benefit of the pilot test was that it helped participants work together to identify common issues and solutions. Through ongoing teleconferences, pilot site coordinators and health records staff from different sites got to know each other. The fact that all sites had access to all the indicator data allowed them to identify sites similar to their own and to bench mark with these other sites if appropriate. A discussion group was set up on the Internet for exchanging information; however, this was not well used by the sites, possibly because not all sites had access to the Internet.

In addition to the teleconferences, education and learning was promoted through a two-day user workshop. An expert from the Center for Performance Sciences in the United States facilitated this workshop. The focus was on how to do appropriate comparative analysis. One of the biggest challenges facing participants was in understanding what it meant when the data were high or low relative to the other organizations. What did the data tell them about their processes? How did they determine whether their organization's performance was satisfactory or whether there were opportunities for improvement? Participants said that this type of learning was invaluable and that the discussions helped them to set up similar education sessions within their own organizations.

Overall, the pilot test provided a stable and reinforcing learning environment in which organizations could gain an understanding about indicator data and develop expertise around using indicator data for improvement. Despite provincial differences, organizations share many of the same issues and learning needs around data quality, comparability of data, and using the data for improvement.

## CONCLUSION

Although the evaluation of the indicators remains ongoing, CCHSA and the participants have gained a greater understanding of the factors that influence the successful use of indicators in an organization. The initial CCHSA visits to the pilot sites, the ongoing teleconferences, and the data quality surveys were all useful. They helped CCHSA and participants understand the issues around consistency of data collection and coding that affect the accuracy and comparability of the indicator data.

The determination of usefulness was more elusive. It was confounded by many factors such as the skill and knowledge of those working with the data, ownership of the indicator data, and the priorities of the organizations. Determining usefulness is an ongoing process that requires identifying these factors and the causal relationship between them.

Whether with these six indicators or any other set of indicators, putting the structures and processes in place to support staff in using indicators is critical to success. Organizations must ensure that there are processes for educating staff about indicators and the role that indicators play in achieving the organization's goals and objectives. Organizations must also be committed to providing the necessary resources for analyzing data and helping team members understand the data. Finally, teams must be able to work toward improvement in an environment that promotes learning in a nonpunitive way.

# REFERENCES

1. Angaran, D. M. 1991. Selecting, developing, and evaluating indicators. *American Journal for Hospital Pharmacy.* 48:1931–1937.

2. Barnsley, J., L. Lemieux-Charles, and G. R. Baker. 1996. Selecting clinical outcome indicators for monitoring quality of care. *Healthcare Management Forum.* 9(1):5–12.

3. Caragata, W. 1998. The high cost of healing. *McLeans.* 111(24):16–18.

4. Maryland Hospital Association, *Performance assessment: the common sense perspective.* 1993. Lutherville: Maryland Hospital Association.

5. Pink, G. H., T. J. Freedman, and Members of the Toronto Academic Health Science Council. 1998. The Toronto Academic Health Science Council Management Practice Atlas. *Hospital Quarterly.*

6. Sutherland, R. W., and M. J. Fulton. 1988. *Health care in Canada.* Ottawa: The Health Group.

# REPORT #4

## THE VIEW AT 30,000 FEET: MEASURING THE PERFORMANCE OF AN INTEGRATED HEALTHCARE SYSTEM

*Arlene N. Hayne, R.N., D.S.N., B.S.N.*

## INTRODUCTION

The building of a system to measure the performance of a healthcare organization requires an extensive understanding of the complexities associated with both the concept of performance measurement and the organization's purpose and structure. The Baptist Health System, Inc. (BHS), located in Alabama, is an integrated healthcare system comprised of 13 acute care facilities, home care agencies, long-term care agencies, senior housing, fitness facilities, a primary care clinic network, and a Health Maintenance Organization with over 300,000 covered lives. BHS has been in the process of designing, implementing, and improving its performance measurement system and its performance at the system level over the last six years.

## CONCEPT AND PHILOSOPHY

The concept of quality in healthcare has been around since the days of Florence Nightingale. When asked about quality in healthcare, many healthcare providers associate their understanding of quality with the term quality assurance. Quality assurance activities historically have been associated primarily with clinical activities in healthcare, regardless of the location of the provision of healthcare. The relationship between clinical performance, satisfaction, and financial performance has only become an area of interest within the last decade. As with any concept, the understanding, scope, and complexity of the concept can only develop over time and research. The concept of quality in healthcare has experienced significant attention over the last decade, resulting in significant documentation and research into various components of the concept. The concept of quality is now associated, not just with the idea of performance measurement, but also with the concept of performance improvement. The concepts of financial and satisfaction indicators are now considered components of the concept of quality. Additionally, the introduction of the theories of continuous improvement and process improvement have been added to the concept of quality in healthcare. Additional understanding of the concept of quality has grown to include the concepts of benchmarking, best demonstrated practice, and most recently, evidence-based practice.

Research in defining, understanding, and measuring quality in healthcare has taken many forms. Scientific studies proving the benefit of certain processes and procedures have been going on for decades and are regularly published in the scientific, medical, and related professional journals. But now, in addition to this type of research, studies are conducted concerning the satisfaction of individuals experiencing those procedures and processes. These studies have developed to include the long-term impact on individuals over time, as measured not just in long-term mortality and morbidity studies, but in functional status studies. These functional status studies attempt to determine how individuals perceive their quality of life following these healthcare events and episodes. Healthcare quality models are also being tested within the healthcare industry in an attempt to better understand the concept and the relationship between the components of the concept. The relationship between various components is also being tested. Cost, outcome, and satisfaction variables are being studied in various settings. In designing a performance measurement system, the designer takes into consideration all of these issues in creating the architecture of the system.

## ORGANIZATION MISSION AND VISION

Likewise, in designing a performance measurement system, the complexities of the healthcare organization, its mission, and its culture must be taken into consideration. The mission of the organization will define to some extent the boundaries and scope of the performance measurement system. The mission of The Baptist Health System, Inc.: "As a witness to the love of God, revealed through Jesus Christ, The Baptist Health System is committed to enhance the health, dignity, and wholeness of those we serve through compassionate care, innovation and performance, education, and research. The core values of health, those we serve, education, innovation, and research represent the key concepts that form the framework to ensure a total organizational approach to quality in every aspect of performance." The BHS believe these core values mean different things to different people. In order for those that BHS serves to be able to evaluate how BHS measures up to other organizations, it is helpful to define core values.

Health is a state of optimal physical, mental, spiritual, and emotional well-being. Attainment requires both prevention and treatment. Health includes a holistic approach which encompasses maintaining an individual's privacy, and treating him or her with respect, dignity, and compassion.

To enhance the health dignity and wholeness of those served is to make a difference or improve the quality of people's lives. Quality is a multidimensional concept comprised of the components of processes and outcomes. Quality processes are specific steps that an organization consistently follows in achieving the required level of performance and include the characteristics of accessibility, acceptability, appropriateness, effectiveness, timeliness, safety, continuity, and cost. Another type of quality processes incorporate continuous quality improvement principles (CQI) and analysis of variances. Outcomes are classified as clinical, satisfaction, financial, or relationships between these variables.

Those we serve are those individuals involved in or served by BHS. There are four categories of those we serve: customers, community, associates, and suppliers. Customers are traditionally inpatients, outpatients and their families, or significant others. Communities are those organizations that represent the payers or major employers of our customers. Communities are also those groups and individuals served by outreach, preventive, or wellness programs. Associates consist of BHS employees and the medical staff. Suppliers are those businesses and individuals that provide goods and services to the organization.

Education is the act of imparting knowledge or skills. It includes patient/family education, staff, community, and student learning. Innovation is the use of new technology or new approaches to doing things. Research is the collection of valid and reliable data that undergo a thorough analysis to be used in decision making.

The environment includes the physical environment, as well as the external and internal social and cultural environment in which the organization finds itself.

From the above paragraphs, the boundaries and scope of the performance measurement begin to take shape. Nevertheless, without executive leadership and commitment, the creation of a performance measurement system of a complex organization will not be successful. The vision of the system executive is a critical success factor for both the integrated healthcare system and the performance measurement system. The senior executive at BHS is committed to BHS being the leading regional healthcare system in the South. He understands the relationship between all of the pieces of the system, how they should work together to create value, and what level of performance will be required in order to achieve the vision of BHS. The synergy that results from the integration activities results in a stronger system that provides a continuum of care and, in addition to point of service satisfaction, actually improves the quality of life for people who live in Alabama. The magnitude of an organization of BHS size and complexity dictates that the resources required to organize, standardize, and improve performance involve a long-term commitment. The president of BHS initiated BHS's commitment to continuous quality improvement at the system level and continues to support it by regular attendance at meetings, allocation of resources, and participation in external improvement reviews, such as the Alabama U.S. Senate Productivity and Quality Award process.

# MODEL

The BHS system level performance measurement system is based on a systems model. Like all systems models, the major components can be defined as processes of inputs, through puts, outputs, a feedback loop, and structures found within the organization. Figure 7.6, The Baptist Health System Inc. Quality Improvement Program System Quality Model, is a one-dimensional illustration of the concept of quality for the organization.

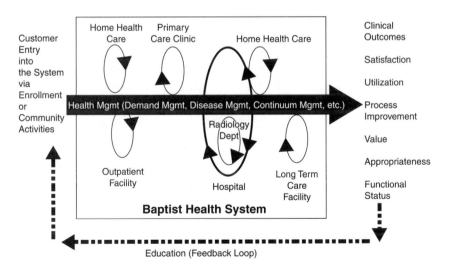

**Figure 7.6.** Baptist Health System, Inc. Quality Improvement Program (QIP) System Quality Model.

The structures include the organization as a system, as well as the individual structures that make up the system. Each of these individual structures, hospital, home care agency, or nursing home is itself a system. All of these structures are comprised of complex processes that occur at the individual employee-customer level, departmental level, interdepartmental level, and across the organizations within the system.

## INPUTS

The inputs into the system are the customers that utilize the services of BHS. The customers can be defined as individual patients, considered as groups of patients, or even the community where BHS provides its services. Defining the customer is important when measuring the outputs of the system. The level of input at the individual, population, or community level provides increased depth and scope to the concept of quality as defined and measured for an integrated health system.

Regardless, if the program or services provided by BHS are directed toward an individual, group, or community, healthcare is accessed one individual at a time. The model illustrates the entry into the health system at one point. Actually, an individual may access a healthcare system at any one point in the organization and move around within a system, from doctor's office, to out patient testing, to inpatient surgery, to home care, doctor's office, and eventually even into a nursing home. It is not a straight one directional path. In the model, it is shown as a one directional arrow to simplify the concept of a health system providing care through the lifetime of an individual, regardless of setting and health status. The use of this model tries to illustrate the interrelationship between the pieces of the system, and the processes within each structure and between each structure. An integrated healthcare system such as BHS, as part of its definition of quality, includes the managing of those processes within each structure and across all processes, because these are the elements that make it a system. The organizations within the system include all of the distinct structures that belong to the system. Because this is a systems model, it would be possible to apply this model at the facility level, with the internal department representing other internal systems and their processes.

## PROCESSES

In the model, *TeamWorks* is illustrated by an arrow depicting process improvement activities occurring within a department, facility, or system.

TeamWorks provides BHS with the philosophy of continuous improvement, defines the responsibility for quality processes and outcomes, and provides the tools to improve the design of systems within departments and organizations, as well as the everyday work processes. BHS began its continuous improvement journey about seven years ago with the introduction of continuous improvement concepts, principles, and tools. Over the last seven years, resources have been dedicated to providing training, dedicated facilitators, and creating teams.

TeamWorks has created a *quality culture* within BHS. This culture emphasizes the importance of understanding and then exceeding customers' expectations, regardless if the customer is a patient, family member, physician, or fellow employee. Using data to understand and control variability is another characteristic promoted in this TeamWorks culture. It also means designing and building systems to do the right thing 100 percent of the time. A continuous improvement organization works in teams to improve its processes and outcomes. Quality work is not something that occurs after the real job is done, but is the way the job is done daily.

Process management and improvement as a methodology taught within TeamWorks includes the steps of focusing on processes, defining a process, analyzing it with the use of flow charts and data, and then improving the process. During the focus stage, it is important to identify and prioritize significant issues, especially as perceived by the customer. Determination of the processes that affect the issues and also who is responsible for managing those processes are critical components of this step. The definition stage is comprised of describing the process, establishing the boundaries of the process, identify standards to be used in measuring the process, and developing or selecting measures to be used in this process. These steps are necessary to reach a common understanding of process flow and appropriate measures, to establish boundaries of responsibility, and limit the process of improvement activity. The next stage, analyze, builds on the previous stages because it uses the measures selected to understand process behavior. It is during this stage that data gathering procedures are designed and implemented, and the process is evaluated for consistency. In the case of inconsistency, determination must be made to establish the reason for the inconsistency, be it special causes or common cause variation. In the fourth stage of process management, measures are taken to enhance performance, acceptability of those changes are determined, and monitoring is initiated to maintain the higher level of performance. The use of this methodology and the accompanying tools of data, flow charts, and problem solving, increase the likelihood that problems will be solved, better systems and processes will be established, and the end result will be greater performance and improved customer satisfaction.

Quality processes and outcomes in the model include the processes encountered as a customer moves through the system and as outcomes resulting from that movement. They can also include quality control processes commonly found within most healthcare organizations. When these quality control processes are included within the understanding of the employee, it reinforces the quality culture, as well as links all aspects of work with quality. Quality control processes may include such processes as calibration of machines, verification of cart or pack contents, expiration dates, and the running of control charts or reports.

Quality processes also include doing appropriate procedures correctly and timely. But at BHS, if the right procedure is done at the right time, with the right equipment, to the right patient, but it is done without love and compassion, the process has not been done right.

## OUTCOMES

Quality outcomes take a variety of forms. Common clinical outcomes relate to mortality or morbidity. The cost of the encounter is considered an outcome of the process. At the department and facility level, key processes and outputs are usually identified as a part of that unit's quality improvement program, and ultimately, part of the facility's program. At the system level, however, that level of detail would recreate a huge and cumbersome program. The magnitude of the details would prevent the system from being able to determine its overall level of performance. At BHS, the individual department, unit, and facility managers are held responsible for the performance of their group of indicators. At the system level, it is necessary to aggregate indicators of performance.

## EDUCATION

Education is a very important part of the BHS systems model of Quality Improvement. Just as using data to analyze and improve processes is a critical characteristic of a quality organization, so also is education. Education that includes the tools and methods described in TeamWorks includes just in time training for teams and facilitator training. But education also refers to continuing education and within a health system usually centers around orientation. Education during orientation is intended to create competent employees that do the right thing every time. Education during orientation also refers to defining expectations of employees as it relates to the quality culture within the organization. The concepts of TeamWorks as well as patient satisfaction are covered during orientation.

Continuing education as a component of a quality health system recognizes that one of the major reasons for doing continuing education is to improve performance. Performance improvement can occur when a new technique or piece of equipment is introduced. But, as evidence based practice illustrates, continuing education should be directed at the performance of care related to the patients found within the organization. The need assessment that is frequently referred to by educational departments unfortunately is rarely tied to the quality improvement program. In fact, the quality improvement program is the identification of educational needs to improve performance. Improved performance is the evidence of the effect of continuing education and improved processes. If this link can be clearly made in the organized quality improvement program, the objectives and direction of all facility education becomes evident and more defensible during budget and staffing reductions.

Likewise, the purpose and function of medical staff credentialing becomes clear when it is incorporated within the facility and system quality improvement program. Performance of the medical staff as it relates specifically to patient care has never been more important to a hospital, clinic, or healthcare system. Moving beyond committee participation to patient outcomes and satisfaction as a means to reappoint physicians to the medical staff will also ensure their interest and participation in the facility quality improvement efforts.

## ROLES AND RESPONSIBILITIES

The TeamWorks philosophy states that everyone is responsible for the quality of the work that they do every day. Responsibility begins with the system board members and includes everyone down to the individual employee.

## BOARD OF TRUSTEE MEMBERS

Board of Trustee members need to know that they are ultimately responsible for the quality of the programs and services provided by the system. They need the knowledge that a system is in place to ensure quality and improved performance. This system has to be comprehensive, systematic, built on appropriate principles and theories, and undergo periodic evaluation. Board members need to be educated about the concept of quality as it relates to the healthcare system and also as it relates to their own performance. At BHS, as part of all new board member orientation, content is included about the system level quality improvement program, their responsibilities, and the concepts associated with TeamWorks. The more board members can be involved in the quality improvement program, the more the organization's quality culture will be reinforced. Given the high level of perspective and decision making that occurs at the board level, it is difficult for true ownership in a performance improvement program to occur. Therefore expectations of Board members need to be reinforced whenever the opportunities exist. Employees at all levels need to hear and read the support of the board members to continuously improve their performance. At the same time, board members can challenge all employees to exceed their customers' expectations. Challenging senior management takes the form of questioning why an organization is at a certain level of performance, if that is the *best* the organization can achieve, and what it would take to get to the next level of performance. The answers to these questions inform board members on how to prioritize and allocate resources. It is imperative that senior management be good stewards of board members' time.

## MANAGEMENT

Management's role within the BHS quality system includes both personal involvement, as well as creating the environment that supports performance improvement. Managers at BHS receive process improvement education and are expected to serve as team champions, as well as members of natural management teams or other interdisciplinary teams. As managers, they are responsible for allocating resources that support the performance improvement activities. These resources can take the form of budget dollars for training, implementing team recommendation, and paying for team celebrations. Management support includes making the necessary arrangements for personnel to participate in teams during work time. Management also has a responsibility to actively participate in the BHS Quality Improvement program by identifying, measuring, and improving critical success factors for their department, including customer satisfaction, process improvements, and outcomes. Participation at the system level may include participation on system level Quality Improvement committees, or serving on ad hoc committees functioning at the system level. Managers also have a responsibility to create systems within their area of responsibility that result in quality processes and outcomes. Communication with employees within their respective departments about quality improvement within their own department, as well as system-wide efforts, is another expectation of managers.

## MEDICAL STAFF

TeamWorks also identifies medical staff members as being responsible for quality improvement at the Baptist Health System. Responsibilities of the medical staff begin with their own individual practice and include serving on facility specific and system level committees. The chairman and chairman elect of the Quality Improvement Congress are physicians. Their role, in addition to leadership of the program, is to define best practice standards and goals for clinical practice improvement.

## EMPLOYEES

Employees, of course, are the linchpin in the entire equation. Quality processes and outcomes have to be performed anew every hour of every day with each patient, family member, physician, or fellow employee. The best designed systems, the most comprehensive education programs, are only as good as the cook in the kitchen, the security guard at the gate, and the nurse turning a hurting patient. Empowering employees to exceed customers' expectations, use process improvement tools, and implement the changes they identify are the processes that really ensure performance improvement.

## STRUCTURE

At the facility level, there has been an evolution from the traditional quality assurance model to a quality improvement model. In some cases, facilities have incorporated the functions of utilization, case management, credentialing, and continuing staff and medical education into the facility quality improvement model. The BHS systems model clearly suggests the benefits of this type of approach. However, facility organization, politics, and maturity will often dictate the model used at the facility level. The important point about the facility model, as it relates to the system model, is that the system model creates synergy throughout the system, prevents redundancies, and builds on the strengths of the individual programs. It is not essential that every facility has exactly the same model and program in place in order for there to be an effective system program. What is essential, is that the system program strengthens and improves the existing programs, thereby improving the performance of the overall system.

## PURPOSE AND OBJECTIVE

The purposes of the BHS Quality Improvement Program (QIP) are threefold. The QIP is to demonstrate improvement in the health of the communities served by BHS; it is to improve the quality of individual lives, both patients and employees; and it is to identify indicators of system-wide performance and value. The objectives of the BHS Quality Improvement Program are to ensure that the programs and services of BHS are the right ones to meet the needs of the individuals and communities BHS serves, and to ensure that BHS continuously improves its programs and services. The BHS Quality Improvement Program does this through planning and organization.

## PLANNING

Planning for the BHS QIP takes two forms, strategic and operational. Strategic long-range planning results in annual system level objectives and in a three-year plan. The strategic planning process is based on the BHS mission and vision statements and aligns system facility and departmental objects with the former. Figure 7.7, BHS Mission Planning and Process Improvement Process, illustrates this process. System strategic objectives are categorized according to integrity, compassion, advocacy, stewardship, and excellence. Clinical and satisfaction performance improvement activities are located within the excellence category. Financial performance improvement activities are found within the stewardship category. Most recently the system level shared objectives included to demonstrate improvement in five system-wide clinical quality indicators, initiate functional status measures, show significant improvement in patient and employee satisfaction, and implement two community health initiatives. These system level objectives are then disseminated to each facility and business unit to be incorporated into their specific objectives. The status of these objectives is reviewed quarterly, and manager's per-

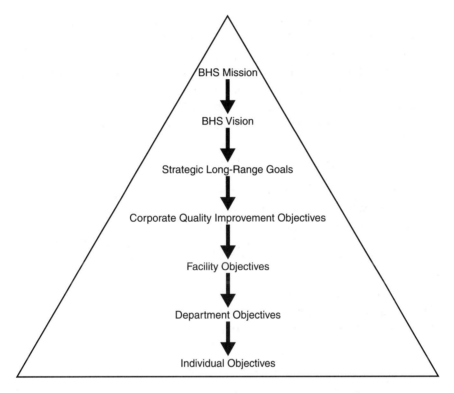

**Figure 7.7.** BHS Mission, Planning and Performance Improvement Process.

formance incentive compensation is tied to the results achieved. This quarterly review is one of the two ways that performance is assessed; the other review occurs through the quarterly QIP reports.

The second type of planning is the strategic and ongoing planning of the QIP. At BHS there is ongoing planning that occurs quarterly through the Steering Committee. This ongoing planning adjusts the program based on feedback from previous meetings and other changes occurring within the organization. Strategic planning for the QIP has occurred once in the six-year history, at approximately the three-year mark.

The purpose of a strategic planning process for the system level QIP was to review the purpose, function, and form of the program; evaluate the effectiveness of the program; and develop a strategic plan for the measurement and improvement of the system's performance. Preparation for the strategic planning process included a review of the annual evaluation results for the three previous years, a summary of the meeting evaluations, a copy of the program description, and the BHS mission and vision statements. Participants at this strategic planning meeting included past and present officers of the QIP, physicians from the regional facilities, and home care representation. Questions the strategic planning process addressed were: Why does this group exist?; What is the work of this group?, including scope, integration, criteria for determination of priorities, definition of terms, evaluation, and goal setting; and How does this group get the work done?, including structure and relationship to other groups and functions. As a result of the strategic planning process, the QIP was reorganized into its current form. The value of this intensive review of a program cannot be overestimated. It is, however, not necessary to do this in-depth review annually, because it is extremely helpful to have several years of data and experience to use in the planning process.

## COMPONENTS

The BHS Quality Improvement Program is organized around three major components: TeamWorks, Satisfaction, and Clinical Quality, which includes case and continuum management.

## TEAMWORKS

The TeamWorks program is structured in such a way that there are trained facilitators at each facility. These facilitators provide *just in time* training for new teams that are chartered for specific purposes. Facilitators can also work with natural management teams to improve the critical processes found within their department, or with cross-functional teams to improve other processes. The use of facilitators and teams is the process that is used to improve the clinical and satisfaction performance of the organization. Individuals responsible for TeamWorks at each facility report quarterly on the activities of their teams.

## SATISFACTION

Customer satisfaction at BHS is comprised of patient, physician, and employee satisfaction. The greatest emphasis is placed on patient satisfaction. Satisfaction is measured at each of the main business units, and managers are held accountable for satisfaction targets. Satisfaction in the

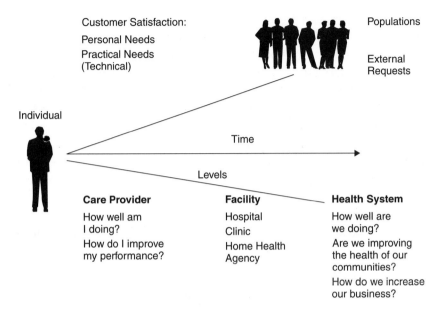

**Figure 7.8.**   BHS Concept of Patient Satisfaction.

acute care areas was, until recently, measured using an internally developed standardized instrument that was administered by phone using an outside agency. This instrument evaluated nursing care, admissions, business office, environment, and physician satisfaction. Recently, the hospitals have begun transitioning to a national survey instrument in order that external benchmarking comparison will be available. Up to this point, the satisfaction measurement program has not segmented satisfaction by case type or population.

Figure 7.8, BHS Concept of Patient Satisfaction, illustrates the evolution of this concept at BHS and shows the relationship between point of service satisfaction and population satisfaction. Point of service satisfaction is a critical component of quality because it measures the outcome of the interaction between each individual patient and the individual employee. Customer satisfaction is related to how well another individual or set of individuals within a unit, office, or during a visit meet the individual customer's personal and practical needs. Personal needs include friendliness, compassion, helpfulness, and so on. Practical needs concern the employee's competence to perform the interaction in an appropriate, safe, efficient, and effective manner. The outcome of this interaction affects the individual patient's outlook of themselves, as well as their experience. This interaction is believed to affect the eventual recovery of the patient and is known to affect self-referral and marketing of the organization. For the employee, it is one of the only ways an employee can receive feedback on their daily performance. And although BHS does not have the mechanisms to track satisfaction by employee, the technology to be able to do this level of measurement does exist.

Point of service satisfaction measures *How am I doing?* but it does not answer the larger organization question of *How are we doing?* in providing care to groups of patients and improving the quality of life for populations found within the community. Functional status measures also enable an integrated healthcare system to evaluate performance over time and across business units. This does not eliminate the need to systematically measure *hands off* satisfaction as part of the continuum; however, functional status measures do aggregate over time the effectiveness of the system's performance as a whole. Functional status measurement also, in an indirect way, can indicate how well an organization is preparing the patient's significant others to support them in dealing with their condition. BHS has no established methods to measure the satisfaction of family members. This level of satisfaction is measured using functional status measures and population measures, such as those found within the Health Plan Employer Data and Information Set (HEDIS). BHS has completed several pilot studies using either the functional status instruments of SF-12 or SF-36 but does not currently have an established system to measuring satisfaction at the population level.

Physician satisfaction is measured annually but only among the urban facilities medical staff. Likewise, employee satisfaction, in the form of a work place audit, is measured annually. Supervisors receive feedback on their results and must submit action plans that address certain response levels, comments, and issues identified in the audit.

## CLINICAL QUALITY

Clinical quality within the BHS Quality Improvement Program consists of two major components: case management and system level performance indicators. Case management activities at the system level focus on the most frequent diagnoses and procedures that occur within the system. These include obstetrical case, congestive heart failure, pneumonia, chronic obstructive pulmonary disease, transient ischemic attacks, stroke, and acute myocardial infarction. System level clinical performance indicators track performance across patient populations and measure the rates of mortality, morbidity, wait time in the emergency department, cancellations of ambulatory procedures, returns to special care or the operating room, and readmission rates. Between the two components, performance involving the care of the majority of inpatient and outpatient populations are evaluated.

## AUTHORITY

The BHS Quality Improvement Program is organized in a manner that attempts to create synergy with existing programs and structures that exist at the facility level, promotes standardization, and maintains the confidentiality and protection from discoverability for litigation purposes. The program description defines the direct link between the system level program and the existing facility quality assurance and improvement programs and restricts communication and distribution of materials within the confines and authorization of those programs. Figure 7.9, BHS Quality Improvement Program Structure, illustrates the structure of the QIP.

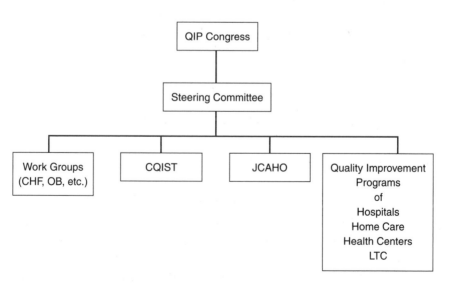

**Figure 7.9.**  BHS Quality Improvement Program Structure.

The BHS Board of Trustees delegates to the president of BHS and to the Quality Improvement Program the authority to establish the system level organization. The president of BHS directs the Divisions, their Boards of Trustees, administrators, and their members to participate in the Quality Improvement Program through their facility level participation, as well as at the system level.

## COMMITTEES

There are three operational levels to the BHS Quality Improvement Program: working committees, congress, and steering committee. Responsibility for the program resides with the corporate director and the elected chairperson and vice chairperson, who are both physicians. Terms of office are for two years, with the vice chairperson automatically assuming the chairpersonship during the second year.

The working committees are comprised of a standing committee and work groups or teams. The standing committee, the Corporate Quality Improvement Support Team (CQIST), has members from all the major business units but consists primarily of hospital quality improvement and case management personnel. Depending on the size and organization of the facility, they may have one or more members attending this committee. The responsibilities of this committee are

- Validity and reliability of data submitted to the QIP
- Submission of data to corporate quality management
- Communication to individual facility departments and individuals
- Sharing resources and expertise in order to accomplish the goals of the program

The JCAHO committee is also a standing subcommittee of the QIP. Representation on this committee is comprised of two individuals from each facility. The patient care services representative and the individual who is responsible for coordinating JCAHO accreditation for the entire individual facility are the two representatives from each hospital on this committee. Other representatives from corporate and the facilities are involved during specific times, depending on the subject matter being addressed.

Work groups or teams are those committees that are not necessarily standing committees. These committees include groups that come together for a specific purpose, meet for a period of time, but may eventually disband. Examples of these work groups or teams include a multi disciplinary committee for the congestive heart failure population or the obstetrical population. Other ad hoc multidisciplinary committees that were appointed included *Door to Needle* time for acute myocardial infarction patients, stroke patients, and emergency department, performance improvement activities.

The QIP Congress is a multidisciplinary, multifacility committee composed of five representatives from each hospital and three representatives from each nonhospital facility and from corporate. The representatives from the hospitals are the president, the physician administrator or chief of staff, a patient care representative, a quality assurance/improvement representative, and the physician chair of the quality assurance/improvement committee. The three representatives from the nonhospital facilities are the facility administrator, the quality assurance/improvement representative, and a physician representative. The corporate representatives are the president of BHS, the Division president, and corporate case management. A conscious decision was made not to include Board of Trustees representation because of the time requirements already placed on board members. However, it would be appropriate to include them in this membership in other systems. Given the size of the Congress, it is too large to be an effective decision-making group. The function of the QIP Congress is to serve as a forum of communication and education about quality improvement within the system. As a communication and education mechanism, it shares best demonstrated practice and internal benchmarking data. It provides the leadership of the system and individual facilities with a broader view of quality improvement. This broader view is critical in designing systems that function effectively across the continuum. Based on the experience at BHS, the ability of participants to visualize quality improvement at this level is difficult. Congress members have to be educated about the value and the methods to examine performance at the system level. System level performance is aggregated to the level that removes it from reality or the ability to actually change a process. Although performance is affected at the individual or facility level, it is these participants who, unless they learn how to see the *forest,* the forest program is of no value. In the early stages of the BHS QIP, a What's in it for me? (WIFM) perspective is all too common. The perpetual defense, *my patients are sicker,* is also difficult to overcome. However, the BHS experience suggests that, with time and education, it is possible to use the Congress forum as a means to share information. After several years of meetings, working together, and education, there appears to be a greater willingness among facility representatives to talk about less than outstanding performance, to want to boast when a smaller hospital outperforms a larger, more sophisticated hospital. This atmosphere is very difficult, if not impossible, to create outside a system because of competitive environments.

The QIP Steering Committee is comprised of representatives from across the system who represent both the continuum of care and information systems. The continuum of care representatives include long-term care, home care, primary care, and acute care. BHS did not include its Health Maintenance Organization (HMO) in the steering committee because of major organizational changes occurring within the HMO. For other systems, inclusion of this group would be logical. Information systems is represented on this steering committee because of their need to understand data needs of the organization and appropriately reflect those needs in their planning and resource allocation process. The responsibilities of the QIP Steering Committee are to advise the Corporate Director of Quality Management and provide oversight to the direction of the program.

## INDICATORS

Within the healthcare industry there appears to be a fair amount of confusion over the terms used to describe elements of performance improvement. The terms indicator, measure, and rate are all used and frequently mean the same thing. In this case, indicator means the description of the measure used to record performance. In most cases an indicator is a rate resulting from a mathematical equation. At BHS, there are three major categories of indicators, two of which are used in the QIP program. The three categories are financial, clinical, and satisfaction. Financial indicators are routinely reported at the system level, as well as the operating unit level. However, the quality assurance laws, which protect peer review information only, do not protect financial information, and therefore financial information is not combined with the QIP information. Financial performance indicators are relevant to the performance of an integrated healthcare system. Determination of the value that the healthcare system provides to the community it serves requires analysis of the relationship between cost, outcomes, processes, and satisfaction. The method of determining this value, however, must be done cautiously in order not to expose the organization to potential litigation.

The choice of indicator's use at the system level is done according to specific criteria. The criteria include the scope of the program itself. In the case of BHS, the scope includes all the care providing facilities of the hospital, long-term care, home care, and primary care. It also includes community health improvement activities, process improvement activities, and satisfaction of those respective areas. It does not include the sports and fitness centers, hospice, and senior housing. The scope and limitations of the BHS QIP program are partially related to manageability of the program, preexisting quality programs, and opportunities to standardize and bench mark. Addition of these other elements will occur as time and resources become available. Within these areas, criteria for the selection of indicators include high risk or problem prone disease or procedure cases. Another criteria selection is the availability and resources required to collect the data. Priority for action on the results of the performance indicators is established by the QIP Steering Committee and based on the analysis of data and the availability of resources. At the system level, it is only possible to work on a few things simultaneously, so prudence dictates the priority. Selection of the clinical indicators results in a multidimensional range of indicators which overlap to some degree. This approach is intended to address some of the issues of appropriateness, utilization, coordination, and risk. The clinical indicators are a combination of case types based on volume and risk, and inpatient and outpatient processes, such as mortality and complications.

The case types BHS chose to measure at the system level were congestive heart failure, pneumonia, TIA/CVA, and myocardial infarction. The indicators for each of these case types included: length of stay, antibiotic administration, ace inhibitor administration, home care referral, readmission rate, and door to needle time. The other clinical indicators that were measured at the system level included selected rates of The Maryland Hospital Association's Quality Indicator Project® (QI Project®), including unplanned returns to the operating room and special care unit, emergency room wait time, cancellation of ambulatory procedures, unplanned readmissions to the hospital, mortality, etc.

Satisfaction from the various groups of service facilities looked at the performance of critical processes such as admission and also at the performance of physicians and nurses.

## DATA SOURCES

Sources of data for a system level performance program, in addition to being valid and reliable, must roll up from the reporting units in order to minimize duplication of effort, as well as be able to replicate the findings and drill down for process improvement actions. BHS has the majority of its hospitals on the same information system which greatly facilitates the collection and analysis of this data. Some information is collected manually through chart review. The more this process can be automated, the greater capacity for analysis, root cause analysis, and problem solving can occur. The maturity of BHS QIP programs included establishment of data collection systems, manual and automated. Four years into the program, as the result of a cost benefit analysis performed by the quality assurance and improvement representatives from all the hospitals, a quality information system was purchased (MIDAS). At this point in the program development, sufficient standardization has occurred that the value of a system-wide information system was obvious to everyone. This is another example of the synergy that can be created when there is a system-wide approach to quality improvement.

## VALIDITY

The validity of the indicators being used to measure the performance of an integrated healthcare system is an important part of any quality improvement program. A discussion of validity is beyond the scope of this article; however, BHS approach to validity was done in the following way. The validity of the clinical indicators was based on the methods used by the QI Project® to establish the validity of the indicators of the inpatient and ambulatory patients found within their data set.

The validity of the case type indicators was evaluated at BHS following two years of measurement of selected indicators. Analysis of the data of these indicators was performed. Second, a review of the literature was done to determine what indicators were being measured outside of BHS. Third, these findings were reported to select physician experts within BHS for review. As a result, several indicators were determined to no longer be valid indicators of performance of the care being provided to these types of patients and were deleted while other indicators were retained.

## RELIABILITY

The reliability of the clinical indicators was established using the conformance assessment surveys that are included with the QI Project® process and the use of statistical analysis that looked for inappropriate values and outliers that may indicate an error in the collection of data. Results of the reliability studies performed at BHS over a five-year period indicated an improvement in the degree of conformity in data collection. The reliability of the case type indicators was never established.

# NEW MEASURES

Given the criteria for the selection of indicators that was described earlier and the need to have data collected over a period of time, changes in indicators are not done easily or frequently. However, evaluation of the effectiveness of the program can lead to a change in the indicators being collected and reported at the system level. Market and environment changes, including the addition or deletion of services, can also create the need for a change in the indicators. The magnitude of resources required to collect data and report it at the system level, as well as the need to limit the sheer volume of reporting, limit the flexibility in adding indicators. It is for this reason that it is not unusual to see where systems use certain indicators as a proxy of overall performance within an organization. The problem with using proxies is that they truly do not represent a sample of performance for that organization. That is why it is important for an integrated healthcare system to have in place a comprehensive program that provides for the appropriate level of analysis and review at all levels of the organization. Aggregate reporting at the system level cannot be intended for evaluation and action unless there is an organization in place that can deal with that level of data.

# REPORTING

## Board of Trustee Reports

Because of the need to be considerate of the amount of time most board members have, as well as the fact that many board members are not in the healthcare industry, the type and amount of information shared with board members has to be succinct, clear, and well organized. At the system level, performance indicates must be rolled up or aggregated. Although the BHS Board of Trustees is responsible for the quality of care provided at BHS, it delegates the function of assessing and evaluating the performance of the system. That function is delegated to the established program. It is the responsibility of the Board of Trustees to create the system and receive reports from the program. At BHS, there are four parts to the quarterly board report. The first part, Figure 7.10, BHS Board of Trustee Quarterly

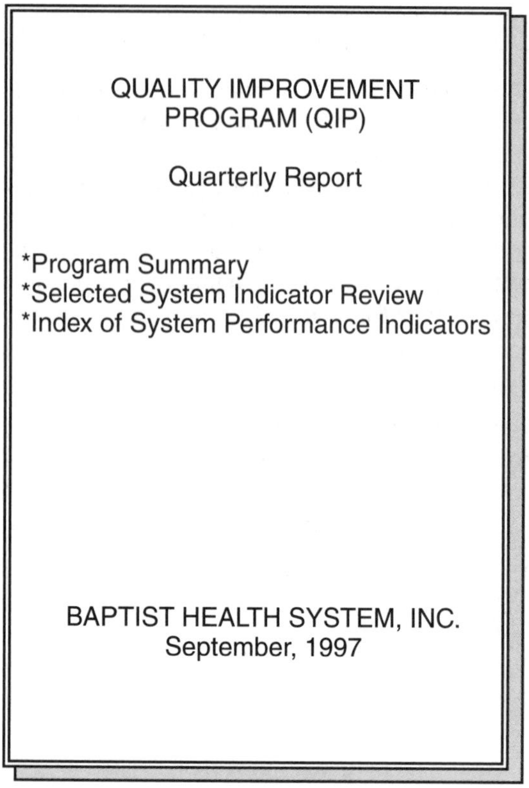

QUALITY IMPROVEMENT
PROGRAM (QIP)

Quarterly Report

*Program Summary
*Selected System Indicator Review
*Index of System Performance Indicators

BAPTIST HEALTH SYSTEM, INC.
September, 1997

**Figure 7.10.**   BHS Board of Trustee Quarterly Report Cover.

QIP Report, is a cover page that also serves as the table of contents. The second page, Figure 7.11, BHS QIP Program Summary, consists of a concise description of the system-level quality improvement program. The purpose of this second page is to educate the board members on the organization and systems that exist at this level to ensure quality. It describes the who, what, when, and why of the quality improvement program. The Selected Indicator Review section of the program summary which follows, is intended to provide a brief education about performance indicators in particular. An example of the narrative part of the Selected Indicator Review is contained in Figure 7.12.

In some circumstances, several related performance indicators are grouped together. For example, when discussing obstetrical indicators,

## Quality Improvement Program (QIP) Program Overview

The Baptist Health System's Quality Improvement Program begins with the alignment of the organization's mission, vision, strategic plans, and definition of clinical quality. Our Mission and Vision Statements provide us with our core values, what we are here to do, where we strive to be, and what we believe and value. Our definition of clinical quality is guided by the Mission and Vision, defined by the organization, and is comprised of standardized components and processes. Standardized quality components are clinical, program, financial, and satisfaction in nature.

### Vision Statement

To demonstrate superior clinical, satisfaction, and value outcomes with continuous improvement to all our customers of health care services.

### Purpose

- Demonstrate improvement in the health of the communities served by BHS.
- Demonstrate improvement in the quality of people's lives.
- Identify indicators of system-wide performance and value.

### Objectives

- To ensure that the programs and services of BHS are the right ones to meet the needs of the individuals and communities.

**Figure 7.11.** BHS QIP Program Summary.

both Caesarean section and vaginal birth after Caesarean section are presented together. In presenting emergency room performance, wait times as well as leaving prior to the completion of treatment are discussed together. This is only logical because of the obvious relation between them. In this part of the board report, the following questions are answered in layperson's terms: Why do we measure this? What does it mean? What are we doing to improve? In answering these questions, external comparative data can be used. This part of the report is the opportunity to engage board members in a discussion using TeamWorks concepts about how to evaluate and improve system performance. This discussion is directed by the senior administrative physician who regularly attends the board meeting.

## Baptist Health System, Inc. Quality Improvement Program (QIP) Emergency Department

*Why do we measure Emergency Department performance?*
In any given year, BHS provides care to over 225,000 patients in our eleven Emergency Departments. For many of these patients and families, our Emergency Department is the very first experience they have with us. Our Emergency Department is a major source of patients for our facilities. An emergency is by definition a crisis in these people's lives and carries "life or death" implications. It is critical then, that our Emergency Departments exceed our patients' and their families' expectations.

*How do we measure Emergency Department performance?*
BHS collects data on the following indicators:

> Satisfaction (Admissions, Nursing, and Physician composite scores)
>
> Door to Drug Time for Acute Myocardial Infarction Patients receiving clot busting drug*
>
> Unscheduled returns to the ED and subsequent hospital admissions within 72 hours*
>
> Emergency Department Wait Times*
>
> Discrepancies in ED X-ray reports requiring an adjustment in treatment*
>
> Registered patients who leave the ED prior to completion of Treatment*

*Participants in external bench marking studies

*What are we doing to improve?*
In February, 1998, BHS QIP held a system wide meeting on these indicators, in order to determine which indicators were the most valid indicators of performance. Discussion at that meeting indicated that satisfaction, wait time and hospital admissions following an unscheduled return to the Emergency Department within 72 hours of a previous visit were indicators with the greatest opportunities for improvement. These indicators will be reviewed again at a systemwide video conference this fall. Every facility has a hospital and Emergency Department committee that reviews this information on a regular basis. At least half of our Emergency Departments have interdisciplinary teams in place actively using the Continuous Quality Improvement process to improve care. This process includes

**Figure 7.12.**    Selected Indicator Review. *Continued.*

reviewing trended data on these indicators. The processes that make up these indicators are flow-charted. Ancillary departments and personnel who own these processes are involved in identifying equipment, education, or different ways to do things which result in either improvement in the process, or innovations to achieving a better result. Examples include posting laboratory and radiology turn-around times in the respective departments, providing quest meal tickets to patients with excessive wait times, and establishing alternative care sites, such as observation beds or medicine clinics.

Satisfaction is collected via monthly telephone surveys conducted by a professional research firm. The survey consists of a sample of 35 randomly selected patients per month per hospital, and uses a standardized survey instrument and scoring methodology. In FY97 there were 4,407 surveys completed, which represents approximately 400 per hospital. Hospitals receive detailed reports on responses to each of the 16 questions in the survey, which have a five point scale response of excellent to poor. In FY98, Princeton and Montclair changed their survey instrument and process, which will not allow comparison to this data. The regional facilities have set goals for improvement in these scores. Satisfaction scores, like all our of performance indicators have to be earned every day with each patient. This indicator is most frequently used as the yard stick of effectiveness of process improvements efforts.

**Figure 7.12.** Continued.

If this administrator is not available to attend the meeting, the chairperson of the QIP, vice chairperson, or the corporate director of quality improvement is present and available to discuss the report. Given the crowded nature of board agendas, it is not unusual for the report to be accepted without discussion. However, it is the responsibility of the senior administrator over the program to take advantage of opportunities as they present themselves to this audience. The final page of the quarterly board report contains an index of all performance measures that are collected, analyzed, and reported at the system level. The purpose of this page is to illustrate the scope of the systematic and organized system level performance improvement program that is in place. No data are given for these indicators, although data are available if requested. The majority of boards do not have the time to receive reports on all of these indicators. That is the responsibility of the Corporate Quality Improvement Council and the quality improvement structures of the respective facilities.

### System Program Report

Reports to the QIP take two major forms: the QIP Proceedings and specific topic reviews. The QIP Proceeding report is published quarterly and is distributed to all Congress members. The content of the proceeding report provides the only consolidated, comprehensive, comparative information on satisfaction and clinical quality performance for the system. The sections of this report are, disease management, home care services, long-term care, health centers, QI Project®, TeamWorks, and satisfaction.

The Disease Management section provides reports on all of the indicators being collected and reported for each type across the system for the most current quarter. Only one data point for each facility for each rate is illustrated. No system means are calculated. The QI Project® section provides three data points per facility, a system year to date mean and standard deviation, an external year to date mean and standard deviation, and goal if available. A system trend is also provided. Not all of the QI Project® rates are provided in the report. The QIP Congress selected which rates were to be reported at the system level, and these are the ones included in the report. The individual facilities have access to all of the QI Project® data, as well as the system data if they need it. Hospital inpatient satisfaction composite scores for nursing, admissions, food services, and room comforts have been reported as year-to-date score as compared to goal. Emergency Room nursing scores are also reported as year-to-date score with goal. As stated earlier, the urban facilities are beginning to use an externally accepted instrument. The results are not adjusted for variation in patient mix or payer class. No overall system satisfaction score or trend is provided in this report, although system results are provided to the Board of Trustees.

The TeamWorks section reports on the formation and activity of all types of teams occurring within the acute care facilities. On occasion, these teams may cross facilities or the continuum of care. For example, a hospital team may be concerned with the rehabilitation of the patients with stroke. Team members may include physical therapy, social work, home health, and skilled nursing personnel.

The long-term care section reports on the performance of both the skilled and traditional nursing units. Although the units have standardized the 15 indicators that they report on at the system level, there is some difference in the definition and calculation of the rates. This report provides three data points for each facility for each indicator; a baseline, current quarter, and year to date. A system mean for that category of long-term care unit is also provided for each indicator.

The primary care centers currently report satisfaction only. Their internal quality assurance activities are reported to their own Board of Trustees. The composite scores that are included in this QIP report are for the interpersonal skills of the physician, the technical capability of the physician, front office impression, access to appointments, and nursing services. Year-to-date results as compared to goal are provided in the aggregate; individual primary care centers are not demonstrated.

Likewise, home care currently only reports satisfaction in the aggregate for all agencies. In the last year, the home care agencies have begun to identify a common group of performance indicators that they will collect data on and report to the system. The satisfaction results in this report are by question and category. The categories include type of services provided, receipt of first visit information, the quality of care, recommendation of agency to others, the quality of nursing, therapy, social, and home care aide services, staff service, medication services, and contact with agency. Only the current quarter results are provided—no trends or goals.

## Special Reports

Specific topic reports are prepared and distributed in conjunction with ad hoc committees and Congress-focused meetings. For example, last spring there was a QIP Congress meeting on *Measuring and Evaluating the Emergency Department's Performance.* Reports were distributed to each facility which showed their performance in all indicators related to the Emergency Department. The indicators from the MHAQIP core set of wait time, returns, unscheduled admissions, X ray discrepancies, and leaving before completion of treatment were included. The National Research on Myocardial Infarction (NRMI) study results for those facilities that participated in that study were included. Satisfaction for the Emergency Department was the final component, along with the number of visits for each department. Where the data was available, system means were also provided. At the Congress, an Emergency Department physician reviewed the system level of performance for each of the indicators, and a panel of administrators, nurses, and physicians discussed their perception of the most valid indicators of performance. Several multi disciplinary teams from different hospitals presented their activities to improve their performance as well. For Congress meetings, regular members were invited, but additional invitations were extended to include all emergency room personnel.

## Report Card

A system level quality improvement program provides a logical platform whenever the discussion of external reporting to the community on a facility or system's performance arises. At BHS, discussion began following the publishing of a *report card* by a local competitive facility. In some other areas of the country, this is a much more sophisticated and complex process. The objective of this effort was to demonstrate BHS's accountability to our mission to improve the health of the communities served by BHS. BHS has little experience in this area and as of this writing has not published clinical performance externally.

The approach used by BHS was to report clinical quality indicators, customer satisfaction, and cost data for the major case types currently being monitored. Those areas, such as medical education and pastoral care, that do not lend themselves to capturing or reporting performance data clearly understood, would be covered in a narrative type of format. The format chosen was to illustrate trends in performance. If there were external comparison or goals available, they were to be included. Within a concise format, definitions were to be included, as well as what activities BHS had undertaken to improve that performance. There had been a task force that pulled together the elements not already included in the QIP; however, the task force was disbanded after a year of work because of budget reductions which eliminated the funds to pay for the publication of a report card.

During the task force activity, the major discussion centered around whether or not to be facility specific. The public's lack of understanding of severity adjusted data was perceived by the task force to be a major stumbling block in the publishing of clinical data. The choice of clinical indicators was related to what had been published in other report cards, both the local publication and what the literature reported. Determination of who would be the real audience of the report card was also a difficult decision. Although originally intended for the lay public and to be included in a newspaper insert, eventually the audience was believed to be the human resource personnel of companies paying their employees health benefits. Obviously the difference in these two audiences is great. Another difficulty experienced by the task force was communicating with all of the internal constituencies within the system. Each business unit that was represented, as well as the areas that were not represented, required communication. Of course the most complex communication plan involved the communication with the medical staff. During the development phase, corporate counsel was also involved to explore the discoverability and liability issues surrounding the publication of this data. It seemed that there was a sigh of relief when the budget was cut, because by then the disadvantages of publishing a report card seemed to outweigh the advantages. Nevertheless, public accountability is inevitable in both competitive markets and managed care environments.

# RESOURCES

## *Staff*

The BHS system level quality improvement program was specifically designed to take advantage of existing programs, services and personnel, and prevent duplication of effort. As a result, the program was staffed with only two employees, a director and a secretary. This department of two was responsible for the collection, coordination, and implementation of the system level program. Coordination occurred with the system structures that were responsible for satisfaction and case management. These departments were staffed with six or more employees. A high level of coordination and integration also had to occur between the facility level quality improvement programs and the system level program.

## *Time Investment*

One of the first efforts focused on creating a communication mechanism, which eventually led to the standardization of certain processes as well as indicators. It was these efforts that led to the ability of being able to report indicators of performance at the system level. Initially, the majority of the facilities were not at the point where they were comfortable using their information outside of their own institution, nor did they see true value in the exercise, only more work. None of the data sources were standardized, and the only data collection process that was standardized was participation in QI Project®. It was only after a substantial investment of time and effort on both their part and the part of the corporate department that the vision could be realized. Standardization of clinical quality data sets and satisfaction instruments took almost two years. It was only after that period that data reporting could begin at the system level. Initially, because the participation in the QI Project® was the most standardized, monthly data points were collected and reported at the system level. This was done in order to have sufficient data points more quickly. If quarterly data points were relied upon, it would have been three more years before the value of system level reporting could be demonstrated. During this same period of time, many of the hospital facilities were also being standardized on a common cost accounting system and clinical data system. Nevertheless, even after five years of effort, manual chart review and data entry is still all too common within BHS. In the last year, a standardized quality management system has been installed in the majority of facilities (MIDAS), which has enhanced reliability and increased standardization and efficiencies across the system. Until all of the data are standardized for each indicator, it is not possible to aggregate the data. If the data are not automated it is very labor intensive to aggregate the data, there remains a high risk for errors, and report preparation is difficult.

Quality improvement data differ from scientific research in several ways. Scientific rigor is usually sacrificed for the pragmatic realities of daily operations, timeliness of data, and amount of data available. Principles of validity and reliability are important to quality improvement data sets, as are sample size. Decisions have to be made concerning the definitions, specifically what is included and excluded from denominators and numerators; how outliers are defined and if they are included; methodology for rate calculations, and so on. However, there must be a trade-off between data and action.

Comparison with external databases is extremely difficult with manual systems. Even before the JCAHO implemented its ORYX initiative, comparison with outside databases required a certain amount of automation and standardization. The value of external comparative databases is their ability to reflect population performance more accurately, and if comprised of patient level data, they are amenable to severity adjustment. Severity adjustment is a critical requirement among physicians. Comparison of their performance with their peers can only be done if the physician is convinced that the patients being cared for are of the same type and complexity. More and more outcome studies have validated the importance of severity in affecting the outcomes of specific patient populations. Comparative databases that still allow for the facility to drill down into their data to the patient level are necessary in order to identify the reason for variation in performance and to design process improvement.

Process improvement activities consistently emphasize the importance of using data to drive decisions. From a statistical point of view, the number of data points and sample size are also critical concepts that need to be understood in using the available data to drive decisions. Depending on the frequency of data collection and reporting, the data points generated may be monthly, quarterly, or in some cases, even less frequent. In the case of semiannual or annual reporting it is very difficult, if not impossible, to obtain sufficient number of data points in order to identify variation and trends. Nevertheless, to implement process improvement activities without sufficient data points may result in inappropriate action being taken.

# LIFE CYCLE

## *Early Successes*

The BHS Quality Improvement Program has been in existence for over five years. In that period of time, the purpose and objectives of the program have been clarified; committees have been established; data elements have been standardized; systems purchased and installed; internal and external benchmarking has occurred; and the program has been used as the vehicle to complete the first multihospital survey with the JCAHO. Early on, a decision was made to begin work with areas that were well established, namely the hospitals. Efforts were aimed at standardizing their indicators and providing them with reports that they could use at the individual facility level but that also indicated performance as a system. The system program thus tried to organize the different silos of care within the healthcare system; hospitals, long-term care, home care, and the primary care centers. No attempt was made to bridge the gap between the silos because of the limited resources available. The concept of continuum management was also just beginning. Once the hospital component was functional, additional work within that component was easier. Standardization of the satisfaction survey was accomplished, and disease management data was a logical addition. The timing of the JCAHO accreditation survey helped to drive the effort of coordination and integration of the hospital component of the system level program. The next step, the choice and purchase of standardized quality management system, was a logical step.

## *Rollout Process*

Once that component was moving forward, attention was given to the long-term care areas. The skilled nursing units and the traditional nursing homes were organized under one corporate officer who was very supportive of the effort to standardize performance indicators. For the skilled nursing unit managers, who were attached to the acute care facility, this was not a new idea. Neither was it to the traditional nursing home managers. However, because the traditional nursing units were not JCAHO accredited, they did not perceive this effort as providing value to them, only more work. As part of the initial effort with this group, it was important to emphasize the use of existing efforts, and then by a process of education, teach them how to more effectively use the information they were collecting. It was not unusual for facilities or units to collect and report data but not to actually improve their processes. The main focus was on collecting and reporting. This is not atypical for many healthcare units and organizations. In that respect, the JCAHO has helped facilities move beyond collecting and reporting to action. One of the ways to get *buy-in* in the early stages is to identify the current process in use to collect and report data. There may be opportunities for the corporate level to provide resources to enhance the existing system. The corporate department began providing each facility and unit with a work sheet for each indicator that they could use to document their actions and was a critical component of their existing quality assurance plan. Likewise, the facilities and units were provided with a report, in the format they designed, to be used in reporting their information to their administration and board. From there it was a logical roll up to show comparative information for the system level.

As the long-term care facilities worked on identifying a common set of indicators, a literature review was also done to determine the availability of benchmarks or industry standards and trends that should be taken into consideration. For example, the emphasis on a restraint free environment in the literature, as well as the availability of studies documenting improvement in the use of restraints, demonstrates the validity of this indicator. Over several meetings, as the group began to work together, there remained an individual or two who continued to resist the effort. The stated reason for nonsupport was that her unit did not have any performance issues that needed improvement. This unit director did not perceive any value with comparing the performance of her unit with her peers, or improving the performance of her unit over the current level of performance. The performance was good enough at the level of current performance. Another form of resistance to the effort came in the form of passive nonparticipation, when a unit manager did not come to any of the meetings. After several episodes of absenteeism, the corporate vice president had to take action in order to obtain compliance. Even after 18 months of effort, these individuals participate physically, but not mentally in the process.

Following standardization of the indicators, definitions, calculations, work sheets, time lines, and initial reports, several months of pilot testing followed. The long-term care group received monthly reports and met every three months. For the first six months there were some adjustments made to the system. Since then the indicators, reports, and so on, have remained fairly constant with only one indicator being added. When the system was operational and the managers acquired a certain comfort level with their data collection and reporting, it was then time to provide *just in time* training for process improvement. In other words, how to use the data becomes the main focus of the process. Using the TeamWorks methodology for process improvement, a trained facilitator from the corporate department of human resource and development provided a training session on the use of data to improve the process. The facilitator was also available to go to any of the units or facilities and work directly with these groups and their data. This is a vital part of the quality improvement program, because without action there is no improvement. Too often, it is too easy to focus on the reports and not the activity that should result from the analysis of the reports. BHS is only just beginning to develop this aspect of the program at both the unit level and the system level.

### Simultaneous Tactics

Over the last five years, the corporate director of the quality improvement program would contact the other major clinical service groups within the system, such as home care and the primary care centers, in order to determine their readiness for participation in the program beyond the reporting of satisfaction. Due to major environmental and organizational climates in those areas, it was not realistic to try and move them forward. However, in the last six months, the home care agencies have demonstrated a readiness to identify standard clinical indicators of performance. Because of ongoing contact and relationship with this group, the corporate director of the QIP was invited to attend. The same steps that were followed in the process of the long-term care facilities and units will be followed in the process of developing the home care agencies. An assessment of what their current state and current needs are will be the first step. Education of what industry standards, the value of comparative data, and how to use the data will be the second major step. The identification of opportunities for the corporate program to facilitate and enhance the work of the agency level program is also an important part of the second step in order to establish communication and trust. Ownership of the indicators and process is the next step, which includes revision and validation of the data sets and reports. Following stabilization of the reporting, training on the use of data with the TeamWorks Process Improvement methodology will follow. This should include taking the training into the individual agency as well.

By working with the department responsible for satisfaction reporting, systems were altered to allow for eventual reporting of patient population specific satisfaction. Pilot testing of the use of the functional test SF-12 was conducted and there was collaboration on the purchase of scanning equipment. Discussions were held on developing correlation studies between the performance indicators of satisfaction and wait time or other indicator combinations. During this time, the system underwent its first multihospital JCAHO survey and received a significantly improved mean score. Application was made for an external review of BHS performance improvement culture, resulting in the awarding of the Alabama U.S. Senate Quality Award.

The approach that has been used at BHS is not the only way to approach a system level quality improvement program. This approach utilized the concept of establishing functional *silos* as opposed to a common denominator across the continuum involving all clinical services. Depending on the maturity, complexity, priorities, and resources of the healthcare system, a different approach may be more appropriate. If the silos are already well organized, standardized, doing internal and external comparisons, then efforts can be directed to identifying improvement opportunities that would link these efforts together.

## EVALUATION

The evaluation of any program is a critical component. One type of evaluation has already been described that occurred during the strategic planning process. For the BHS QIP, however, there were two other types of evaluation that occurred. The first type of evaluation was the meeting evaluation. Following each Congress meeting, participants were asked to complete a one-page evaluation form. This form provided feedback on the process of the meeting, as well as the content. This evaluation also was required in order to assign continuing education credits to the sessions. The second type of evaluation that was done was the annual evaluation. This evaluation has taken two forms over the years. One format was a survey that was sent to all members of the Congress that requested feedback on the importance or relevance of each indicator to their facility and the ability of the indicator to be improved. Questions also asked about the form, frequency, and content of the meetings and reports. A second type of evaluation has been used once and consisted of the use of an outside survey company to perform a telephone interview of all the members of the QIP Congress. The questions included in this survey were less about the individual indicators and more about the structure, focus, and value of the QIP.

The effectiveness of the BHS QIP is measured against the purpose and objectives of the program. The purpose of the BHS QIP is to demonstrate improvement in the health of the communities and the quality of individual lives. Analysis of the indicators suggests that performance has improved in certain indicators, remained the same in others, and in some cases deteriorated. The performance indicators that have improved are in many cases those indicators where facilities and the system have focused improvement efforts. Another purpose of the QIP is to identify indicators of system-wide performance and value. The program has and continues to do so, as evidenced by the index of performance indicators for the system which numbers ninety. The QIP now has an organized approach to measuring and evaluating the performance of the system for many of its critical areas. There is a Board of Trustee orientation component which reviews their accountability for quality improvement and the system in place at BHS. There are quarterly reports to the Board of Trustees comprised of standardized indicators which represent the major lines of business. There is integration of the facility programs, as well as system level multidisciplinary, physician driven activities to improve clinical performance for BHS major populations. The integrity of the QIP is assessed and revised regularly based on reliability studies, annual evaluations, and external reviews. The establishment of system level goals has met with mixed results. The process of setting goals was initiated several years ago following a Congress review of obstetrical indicators. At that time, each facility was directed to return to their medical staff, review their data, and determine facility specific targets of improvement. As a result of this effort, the majority of facility performance improved resulting in an overall system level performance improvement. However, the establishment of a performance improvement target for selected indicators of case types based on facility improvement over baseline was not effective. Facility performance did not improve, resulting in no system level performance improvement.

Consistent with these forms of evaluation is the *State of Quality* report provided at the system level strategic planning session, which summarized the five years of activity of the QIP. The State of Quality report was intended to review BHS performance as measured by the indicators reported at the system level and discuss opportunities to differentiate BHS performance in the future. A historical perspective was included in the form of bullet points identifying major land mark accomplishments occurring at the system level over the last 10 years. The analysis was performed by indicator set for each service area. Each indicator set was analyzed for validity and reliability, and concepts of statistical process control were applied looking for common cause variation. Consequently, the determination of goals, availability of external standards or benchmarks was determined, and the current level of performance was assessed. Issues addressed in the report included community health measures, lack of severity risk measures, publication of the external report card, linking of satisfaction with outcomes by specific patient populations, and demonstrating functional status improvements. Using frequent and varied types of evaluations during this process has resulted in major changes in the QIP effort. However, after almost six years of work there remains substantial work to be done to effectively move a system of BHS size forward.

## LESSONS LEARNED

The lessons and experience at BHS during this time are not unique to the experience of other healthcare facilities and integrated health systems. The most essential element is that of executive commitment and support that is clearly and frequently stated and demonstrated through personal commitment and resource allocation. Education of everyone is also a major ongoing requirement of a system level program. Coordination of effort is necessary to prevent duplication and build on the best of what is currently available. Facilitation is also a major characteristic of a system level program of quality improvement. By facilitating the work occurring at the department and facility level, the individual responsible for performance improvement at the facility receives the benefit of assistance from the corporate level. In other words, they receive local benefits for their efforts to contribute to the system program. Coordination, facilitation, and education all require a great deal of communication, and it is communication that has to occur regularly, frequently, and be geared toward the level of the recipient, be they Board of Trustee or department level employee. Communication includes not just the existence and purpose of the system level program, but also the concepts of quality, satisfaction, and continuous improvement, as well as the tools and methods to improve performance. The other major requirement for the successful development and implementation of a system level performance improvement program is perseverance. Any project of this magnitude takes a significant amount of time, resources, and commitment. As evident from the description provided in this account, six years of effort have resulted in functional data systems and improvement processes. However, the magnitude of what remains to be done means that persistent major efforts must continue.

# 8

# Reflections on the Past, Present, and the Future of Performance Measurement

It used to be fashionable for clinicians to say "my patients are different" or for administrators to say "I have an institution to run and I do not have time for quality." These statements reflect outright opposition within the health-care system to the quantification of performance. Typically, such responses become even more vehement when claims are made that a *single method* to measurement can paint a complete and accurate picture of quality. Quality has, for perhaps understandable reasons, usually been associated with the performance of the clinician. Indeed, in the 1980s, and 1990s health services research primarily concentrated upon the measurement of the clinician's decision making, contrasting his decision-making with that recommended in the printed media or by various professional associations. The futility of this exercise has not been universally accepted, even though the placement of the clinician at the center of the provision of care may not be the best approach to performance assessment. The clinician's performance has often been considered to be more of an art than a science. Moreover, the scientific quantification of performance now involves not only the clinicians' performance, but the performance of payers and institutions as well. This is a fundamental trend that we believe will continue in the beginning of the next millennium. The successful design and evaluation of a performance measurement system are functions of our ability to understand the environment within which they are applied. A performance measurement system is based on a systematic approach to measurement which describes clinical decision making and the application of existing science to the ailing patient. Recently, the performance measurement system has been viewed as incomplete if it does not extend measurement throughout the continuum of care.

In the 1980s, performance measurement systems relied on indicators, primarily *quality* indicators. During that period, a number of national initiatives successfully demonstrated that indicators can point to areas worthy of further investigation, eventually leading to quality improvement. These initiatives also demonstrated that indicators do not directly measure performance in its totality. Rather, they measure some aspects of performance that need to be supplemented by other measures to provide a picture of performance that includes all its major components: quality, access, cost considerations, and satisfaction of the participants. While, by definition, incomplete, many of these indicators have served as screens to help users evaluate healthcare. A decade later, our ability to understand and apply performance measures has considerably improved. Today, throughout the world, experiences with performance measures have been shown to be replicable and amenable to scientific scrutiny and societal evaluation.

How do we establish an evaluative framework for a performance measurement system? The literature is filled with recommendations regarding independent dimensions of performance processes and outcomes associated with performance. In this book we presented a model with an operational framework that unifies recommendations from the literature on performance assessment and quality improvement. This model expands definitions of quality and epidemiology and recognizes subjectivity in the equation of performance measurement. It is an interesting development, we believe, that includes both objectivity and subjective expectations from the patients and the provider in the same model. We have emphasized the need to include multiple dimensions of performance in developing useful approaches to its measurement. The experience from the field is clear: state-of-the-art performance measurement involves a consideration of social and individual values—a point we stressed in our operational model of performance.

## Speculation in an Era of Rapid Change

Performance measurement is becoming increasingly sophisticated, in part, due to advances in its understanding and conceptualization, progress in the science and technology of measurement, and advances in the technology of data processing. Yet, with this increased sophistication, there remains concern about the current ability to compare performance among healthcare organizations in a scientifically rigorous manner (Iezzoni, 1997). It seems likely that the future of healthcare performance measurement hinges as much on the evolution of healthcare as it does on the evolution of the discipline of performance measurement.

To even begin to speculate about the future of performance measurement in healthcare, one has to ask the question: What will healthcare look like in the future? This question suggests yet another series of questions: What future? Is the future three years, five years, or ten years? If the past is any guide, the future will be here sooner than we think. In that same vein, we may overestimate the amount of change that will occur in the next two or three years and underestimate the change that will occur in the next ten years.

Although there are few absolutes in healthcare, Roper (1997) indicates that the movement away from individual fee-for-service medicine appears certain, although this too may have its limits. Perhaps less than certain but at least highly probable is the movement toward increased integration of health services and systems. Other scenarios that are likely include continued movement away from inpatient to ambulatory care, increased *portability* of health services and information, more services geared toward an aged population, increased emphasis on primary and secondary prevention, increased collaboration between medicine and public health (Lasker, 1997), and greatly improved health information through the use of large databases. It is also likely that there will be increased emphasis on addressing the appropriateness of care (Naylor, 1998).

Advances in human genetics research are likely to play a huge role in healthcare early in the next millennium. The most widely publicized work in genetics research is the Human Genome Project, a 15-year effort coordinated by the U.S. Department of Energy and the National Institutes of Health that was begun in 1990. This Project has four main goals: to identify all the estimated 60,000 to 80,000 genes in human DNA, to determine the sequences of the estimated 3 billion chemical bases that make up human DNA, to store this information in databases, and to develop tools for data analysis (U.S. Department of Energy, 1997). Results of this work could lead to a radical shift in medical screening and treatment that will lead to mainly preventative approaches to healthcare in the future. Such a shift in approaches could have a dramatic impact on performance measurement in healthcare since the criteria of good and bad performance would change substantially from current criteria.

Despite our prognostications about changes in healthcare, the impact of these changes on performance measurement is as uncertain as the specifics of those changes themselves. One thing is clear, however: the application of performance measurement has, as yet, to match the sophistication of the available technology of information systems. The computer power is there; the ability or will to collect, synthesize, and report data with high levels of accuracy is still not universal. Until it is, or is nearly so, valid performance measurement in the healthcare arena will continue to suffer.

### Developing a Gestalt of Performance

The ability to develop global measures of organizational quality—to develop so-called lists of *good* and *bad* performers or *four star* ratings—is seriously limited. Performance is still viewed and measured in a piecemeal fashion in the healthcare arena. Segments of performance content (surgical infection rates, CABG mortality, Cesarean section rates) are broken out, dissected, and counted. While this approach is useful in identifying specific areas most in need of quality improvement, no total picture of performance, no *gestalt,* emerges out of these piecemeal attacks, regardless of what current performance measurement system is applied. It is not likely that the development of more performance indicators, coupled with the refinement of existing indicators, is going to lead to any substantial change in this situation. The main reason is that a myriad of performance measures already exists, and these measures probably cover just about everything that can be measured in healthcare organizations.

Why is it necessary to develop a performance *gestalt?* One reason is that health plans, indemnity insurers, regulatory agencies, and consumer groups are clamoring for comparative information on performance. What they are likely to receive—if, in fact, they receive anything at all—is a medley of measures of cost and *quality.* Cost data are better understood, more accurately quantified, and easier to gather than quality data, and, not surprisingly, they often take precedence over quality data. In determining *value,* which is directly related to quality and inversely related to cost, cost is therefore more likely to be the major consideration. Since there is often a trade-off between cost and quality, this approach can have a compounding deleterious effect on quality.

*If performance is to be measured in any global sense in healthcare, what may be needed is a change in tactics—a paradigm shift, if you will (Kuhn, 1962).* If and when this new paradigm will arrive and how it will be structured is anybody's guess. However, there are some hints—gleaned mostly from twentieth-century developments in other disciplines—as to how a new paradigm might develop and what form it will take.

## PERFORMANCE MEASUREMENT AND DARWINISM

Most discussions about *quality of care* fail to go beyond considerations of definition. One of the most recent and frequently cited definitions of quality of care was proffered by the Institute of Medicine (Lohr, 1990). Their definition of quality is *the degree to which health services for individuals and populations increase the likelihood of desired health outcomes and are consistent with current professional knowledge.* While definitions abound, there is a dearth of theory, or at least, a dearth of well-developed, competing theories in the areas of quality and performance as these constructs pertain to healthcare. There is presently little theoretical competition with the structure-process-outcome model offered by Avedis Donabedian (1980).

The history of scientific advancement portrays a Darwinian picture: many theories are born but only the most fit survive. For the most part, those theories that survive are heuristic by nature—perhaps dying but in the process giving birth to new, competing theories. Competition in the Darwinian jungle of ideas is absolutely essential to the development of a legitimate science. To draw on an example from psychology, how would the study of *personality* have fared in this century if discussions focused only on definition and Freud's psychoanalytic theory? Freud was a giant in early psychology whose theory, while perhaps not verifiable in a scientific sense, spurred the development of other ideas and competing theories which could be studied scientifically. Nonetheless, reliance on the conceptualizations of Freud would have seriously curtailed advancement of the scientific study of personality during this century. Freud's formulations, however brilliant, did not give direct rise to the science of psychology—to its rigorous experimental methodologies and to the technologies of individual measurement.

*Despite underlying similarities in the factors that contribute to the scientific advancement of various disciplines, there have been identifiable differences in their characteristic reasoning processes.* For example, in medicine, the process of induction—reasoning from particulars to a general conclusion—appears to have predominated. A case in point was the finding that good hygiene (especially rigorous hand-washing) was associated with lower hospital infection rates and mortality in hospital maternity wards during the nineteenth century. The discovery of this association was a backdrop for the development of germ theory. In the social sciences, the process of deduction—reasoning from the general to particulars—has been predominant. This emphasis on deduction has led to the development of a rich assortment of theories and a science capable of accurately measuring individual differences or *qualities.* This emphasis, strangely enough, has not led to any sort of consensus; theories abound with predictions that are at clear odds with one another. For the most part, those models and theories with long-term survival do the best job of explaining the data or what we directly experience through our senses. Once again, we return to the *Darwinian nature* of science.

Science benefits most when both reasoning processes, induction and deduction, are used—even though the latter, to some extent, appears to be more efficient. We believe that what is most beneficial to science is also most beneficial to performance measurement. *The developers of future performance measures must be aware of the power of both types of reasoning processes but must be especially attuned to the need for theoretical advancement.* Such advancement is contingent on hypothesis development and testing, in short, on deductive reasoning.

## PERFORMANCE MEASUREMENT AND THE POLITICS OF THE FUTURE

There is little in this world that remains unaffected by politics, including performance measurement in healthcare. Politics not only plays a role in performance measurement, it plays a major role. There are probably only a few areas in performance measurement in which politics are not involved or at least have no major involvement. The actual science of measurement—its mathematical and statistical basis—is independent of politics. Perhaps the information systems, or at least their architecture, are independent of politics. The *scientific assessment* of performance measurement systems, their reliability and validity, is or should be independent of politics. Beyond these few domains, we are hard-pressed to come up with arenas in performance measurement where politics do not play a major part.

Perhaps the area where politics most directly impact performance measurement is in the fiscal arena. Both public and private sources are responsible for *political* decisions about funding basic and applied research initiatives in performance measurement. At the institutional level, hospital executives make political decisions about the funding level of quality assurance departments, which depend on performance measurement systems for information. How performance measurement fares as a funding priority is determined by a multitude of factors. These include the belief that performance measurement will help institutions improve their performance and better manage their institutions; mandates from accreditation, licensing, and other regulatory agencies; and the level of demand for such information from payers, consumers, and the public, in general.

Future improvements in performance measurement are heavily dependent on sustained if not increased levels of funding for research. In turn, the level of funding will be determined by the actual and perceived success of performance measurement systems in supplying healthcare professionals, accreditation agencies, payers, and consumers with useful information upon which to base decisions about healthcare. For example, if the development of large databases for performance measurement is to be funded, the performance information gleaned from these databases must justify the costs of their development and maintenance. For this and other reasons, it is difficult to make a prediction that large databases will become an important instrument of medical quality improvement in the near future. Davidoff (1997) in a recent article appearing in *The Annals of Internal Medicine* suggests that the future of such databases may be determined as much by "social and emotional forces that govern the diffusion of all innovations as by the technical strengths of databases themselves."

## MEASURING IMPACT

*Ultimately, it appears that performance measurement systems will fail or thrive on the basis of their demonstrated impact on performance.* To date, there are only a few studies that demonstrate the effectiveness of performance measurement in improving outcomes of healthcare (Kazandjian & Lied, 1998). Technically, most of these studies rely on correlational evidence, so that it may be more proper to state that they demonstrate an *association* of performance measurement with improved outcomes.

There are probably a number of other reasons for this dearth of evidence of the impact of performance measurement on improving outcomes. First of all, such studies require some form of cohort analysis—following the same group over a period of time—coupled with a control group. Finding a suitable control group may be even more problematic than following a cohort long enough to demonstrate impact. Moreover, most of these studies do not fit the strict requirements of experimental design. Rarely is there random assignment of subjects to conditions—one of the primary requisites of experimental design. Approaches based on matching control and case groups are often flawed in the sense that there is inadequate matching of populations on all characteristics related to outcomes; in addition, attempts to adjust for differences in the populations may not be completely successful.

### Medicine or Social Science

The development of organizational performance dimensions—including in them the expectations of both recipients and providers—signals a fundamental change in our understanding of medicine. Our recommendations include looking at medicine as a social science, rediscovering medicine as a social science, and placing the provision of care within the dimensions of social expectations. Using multidisciplinary concepts and methods in building performance models, we believe, is a step in the right direction. The rediscovery of medicine, its sociology and anthropology, is not just an academic exercise. What was once believed to be fact-based research, such as the development of clinical protocols and establishing thresholds for acceptability in the decision-making process of clinicians, is now viewed as utopic, incomplete, and academic compared to a multidisciplinary approach to performance measurement. Moreover, in our view, the pursuit of a set of guidelines based on consensus criteria has not been completely successful. The reasons for this encompass regional variability, community expectations (that have to be taken into account in the adoption of any set of performance measures or criteria of appropriateness), and the moving target of medical and sociological knowledge.

Performance is a complex concept and its operationalization demands methods that are portable across systems and are consistent with the current state of knowledge. We believe it is important to establish a baseline of community expectations in healthcare. By *community,* we are referring to all members of a group of individuals that reside within a well-defined geopolitical area. Establishing a baseline of community expectations has implications for measurement and evolution as well as the public presentation of data. Such an approach can benefit from the models used in epidemiological research investigating the prevalence or incidence of phenomena. In this case, we propose the establishment of the prevalence profile (which encompasses rates and numerator data), an approach that follows the first step of any epidemiological inquiry.

Second, we believe it is critical to identify the epidemic. By *epidemic* we mean *what befalls upon the people,* its original meaning. In this case we are talking about the extent and value of social services and the ultimate good that is provided through medicine. This is the concept of the epidemiology of quality (Kazandjian, 1995). Unfortunately, the *epidemic* can also refer to the provision of services that results in unacceptable or unanticipated outcomes or that have adverse consequences on the financial system supporting healthcare delivery. For these reasons, the understanding of what constitutes an *epidemic* of bad quality or dys-quality becomes a second stage in our investigative strategy.

Following the establishment of this somewhat unique way of looking at the concept of an epidemic, we need to consider an investigative process which borrows many approaches from the industrial field of continuous quality improvement. This investigative process uses industrial tools and methods and borrows from the industrial philosophy regarding the process of service delivery, identifying variations, identifying the common cause variations, and identifying exceptions to rules. Again we suggest that focusing upon the physician alone is unacceptable and obsolete. Teamwork and the team concept are paramount in the provision of care, even though the clinical dimension is a critical component of care.

We have demonstrated that dimensions of performance cut across departments or services within an institution, and, more importantly, that these dimensions must include the patient's and the community's expectations. Focusing upon the institution alone, no matter how validly and reliably described, is an incomplete and misleading approach to performance measurement.

We have proposed that it is invalid, given the knowledge we have accumulated in the past 20 years in health services research, to focus only upon an institution or an individual provider as the unique and definitive representatives of the healthcare system. Further, we have demonstrated that expectations, given the current state of knowledge of both the provider and the recipient, cut across the continuum of care. It is not only the application of biological sciences that contributes to the amelioration of health status of people in communities, but also the humanness of healthcare providers contributing to the perception by the recipients that they have encountered responsive and responsible service from their providers. The dissemination of valid performance data to both public and private agencies as well as consumers can be hugely beneficial to society—something that the new technology, such as the Internet, has made possible. Nevertheless, without an accurate and clear representation of comparative performance data, widespread availability of *performance information* will not ensure long-term societal benefits.

We have tried to demonstrate that performance measurement can be compared to the study of anatomy. In fact, it could be said that outcome measures and indicators are the anatomy of performance. These are the observable manifestations that are the starting point for our decision to investigate and learn about causative factors. Our goal is more in tune with gross anatomy than it is with physiology. That goal can best be achieved through a detailed understanding of the multidimensional and highly correlated processes of performance. Then we have to map the various paths, routes, obstacles, and nexuses along the way of delivery to agree on the best care and caring through the best science at a price affordable and acceptable to the community. Until then, we continue our search for performance models that are based on sound epidemiological and social science principals and methods, performance models that reflect current and future realities and possibilities in healthcare.

## REFERENCES

1. Davidoff, F. 1997. Databases in the next millennium. *Annals of Internal Medicine.* 127(8):770–774.

2. Donabedian, A. 1980. *Explorations in quality assessment and monitoring. Vol. 1. The definition of quality and approaches to its assessment.* Ann Arbor: Health Administration Press.

3. Iezzoni, L. 1997. The risks of risk adjustment. *JAMA.* 270(20):1600–1607.

4. Kazandjian, V. A, ed. May 1995. *The Epidemiology of Quality.* Aspen Publishers, Inc. (1996 Best Sellers List)

5. Kazandjian, V. A., and T. R. Lied. 1998. Cesarean section rates: effects of participation in a performance measurement project. *Joint Commission Journal on Quality Improvement.* 24(4):187–196.

6. Kuhn, T. 1962. *The structure of scientific revolutions.* Chicago: University of Chicago Press.

7. Lasker, R. D. 1997. *Medicine and Public Health.* The New York Academy of Medicine.

8. Lohr, K. N., ed. 1990. *Medicare: a strategy for quality assurance.* Washington, D.C.: National Academy Press.

9. Naylor, C. D. 1998. What is appropriate care? *New England Journal of Medicine.* 338(26):1918–1920.

10. Roper, W. 1997. *The new environment for health services research: private and public sector opportunities.* AHSR presidential address. *Health Services Research.* 32(5):549–556.

11. U.S. Department of Energy Publication. *Human Genome Program Report.* Oakridge National Laboratory: Office of Energy Research and Office of Biological and Environmental Research, November 1997.

# Index